Brain Self Care

2 books in one: Stranded Brain and Listening To My Body - Unlock your brain's healing potential to manage stress, become more productive and improve your brain power

By Dr. Belinda Hollis

Stranded Brain

Introduction to Neuro Linguistic Programming

How to Stop Overthinking, Quit Procrastination Mood, Start Positive Inclinations, and Gain the Self-Esteem to Say "Yes"!

By Dr. Belinda Hollis

Introduction

Overthinking is an issue which has plagued humans since the first people had brains. Now as time has moved on and our culture and technology has begun to move at an ever-faster pace, it has become all the more common. We are constantly finding ourselves compulsively checking our phones to see what kind of praise or vitriol our social media posts have gained. This fast-paced society we live in makes overthinking all the more easy in that we now find ourselves worrying about more nebulous threats than the lion that's chasing us. Our concerns now deal more with issues that we cannot directly confront such as bills, grades, marital problems, etc. It can seem impossible to ever get some downtime and truly unplug from this chaotic world

We are all familiar with the uncomfortable feeling that stress can bring us and how it can damage things like our heart and our sleep. But few of us have perhaps ever sat down and wondered how we can combat this too common ailment.

This book has been designed in written to help you combat and understand how overthinking works. A simply written and easy to understand guide on how you can prevent overthinking and what causes it. From the way that overthinking can clutter your mind and make any and every decision seem incredibly challenging, to how negative influences and bad habits can lead to more overthinking.

Often times when people try to go about understanding and then defeating overthinking, they miss one of the most important components of defeating anything, and that is to know your enemy.

With multiple sections on what can cause overthinking in this crazy world. You will find that after reading through this your understanding of overthinking will go from a simplistic world view. To one that allows you to see and understand all the nuances associated with it. As a result, you will quickly be able to combat many of the issues associated with too much thought, such as lack of sleep, poor mental health and most importantly the negative physical health that can incur. Speaking of poor sleep, an often-overlooked part of overthinking is how negative and poor sleep can affect your mental health. Well, this book has a whole section dedicated to trying to get the right amount of sleep when you need, and how to break many of the negative sleep habits that develop in our world today.

Finally, this book will conclude with a deep discussion on meditation and its effectiveness in treating overthinking. It will teach you from the basics such important topics as: how to meditate, where does meditation come from, and how it can defeat overthinking. By utilizing all of these different methods in conjunction with each other you are now setting yourself up to be in a scenario that will allow you to combat overthinking in the most efficient way possible. All while being simple and easy to understand. Now you will have the tools to defeat overthinking. With these tools at your disposal, you can finally begin to live the happy and amazing life that you very much deserve.

Before going any further, I want to thank you for choosing this book and, if you enjoy it, make sure to leave a short review on Amazon, as I would love to hear your feedback.

Chapter 1: The Basics of Overthinking

In short overthinking can best be described as putting too much thought into issues that perhaps do not require a whole lot of thought to begin with. Take for example someone who worries constantly about how they will pay their bills, they tend to be under the assumption that by worrying about paying their bills they are somehow working to fix the problem.

The reason for assuming this makes quite a lot of sense, if you assume that most problems can be fixed with brute force and a lot of cognitive input. It becomes easy to assume that by constantly thinking and thinking about said bills that perhaps you will be able to pull a rabbit out of the hat and then go about solving the issue. This while seeming like a helpful way to solve a problem is in fact quite counterintuitive.

For the simple reason that there are some problems that require nothing but time to fix. As a result of this shift in how our problems are viewed now people often find themselves in this trap of constantly worrying about an issue even if said worrying is not going to do them any good. This is because we as humans love to feel like we are in control of a situation even when we are not, by constantly thinking about something we can gain this illusion of control.

When we overthink in the hopes of gaining this elusive control, we may start to find ourselves in a worse off spot then we began. This is because overthinking as a trait is very good at tricking us into feeling worse about a situation then we should. Our thoughts go from being focused on solving a problem to worrying about other issues that are unconnected, our mind becomes a torrent of what if the how's is, and the why's.

Instead of simply accepting that perhaps we have no control over the situation. Distress likes to rear up when we start behaving like this, we begin to spend all our time worrying in our heads about some nebulous threat that is abstract and hard to pin down. We lose sleep which then ends up furthering our negative mental state. In many ways overthinking is a very cyclical behavior we start worrying about worrying, in short, we fear, fear. Overthinking does not just have to be a series of thoughts about paying rent or getting our car payments done.

Often times the most commonplace that we can find overthinking is in our day to day interactions with people. People who overthink can find themselves in many different social situations where they begin to spend an inordinate amount of time worrying about every little interaction they have and how people begin to think of them. This can prove to be extremely damaging as instead of just being our true selves we begin to try to tailor ourselves to the unchained ideas that we have in our mind.

When I say unchained what I am referring to is the fact that most of our worries and fears that arise from overthinking, are in fact highly irrational and have no basis in reality. Yet they feel very real, it's easy to believe every single thought that bounces around in your head. Because we all like to have this assumption that most of our thoughts are true and correct but this is simply false. Most of our thoughts tend to come from a place of emotion and we then justify them with logic.

So how can overthinking affect you? Well, the most common way that overthinking can begin to show its negative effects is in the manifestation of psychic tension, better known as anxiety. Anxiety is defined as a persistent state of worry and fear usually over trivial things. This anxiety can slowly begin to build up to the point where it will begin to affect us in our day to day lives. This fear almost always begins from the act of overthinking. We start by assuming that what we are doing is of some benefit to us, from there we then move on to a stage of persistent fear and worry.

When someone is constantly worrying and in fear, they begin to lose sight of things. Instead of focusing on their job or their partner and the like. People now begin to find that their time has begun to be primarily preoccupied with various fears and worries.

This can start to manifest itself in a physical way. I am sure you have heard of people who worry so much they give themselves stomach ulcers or have panic attacks. Think of it simply like this overthinking is mostly caused by excess mental energy at a certain point that energy has to go somewhere. At some point that energy will be redirected to the body. This is where overthinking truly becomes bad when it starts to actually harm us physically. On Top of causing various bodily issues overthinking can harm are sleep. When we are trying to get to sleep, we should not have our mind running a million miles a minute instead we should be calm and allow ourselves to slowly drift off to sleep.

Lack of sleep as well as being very annoying. It is also very bad for our mental health. When we do not get a whole lot of sleep, we can actually find yourself thinking more than we normally would thus perpetuating this already irritating cycle. Instead of getting to sleep peacefully we can find yourself staring at the ceiling while an innumerable amount of pointless thought starts to cloud our mind and we begin to lose sight of what we should actually be doing. In concluding this section, it is important to remember that while overthinking can seem like a helpful thing for us to do. It is in fact quite counter-intuitive to how we are designed. Simply put our brains are not designed to be constantly filled with pointless thoughts. While, yes, we are designed to think and use our brains. We are not designed to constantly be thinking about pointless things that we cannot change. This may be hard to accept but if you can accept it you will be better off as a result. Once you can quit overthinking you can put your cognitive powers to better use than just simply worrying all the time about things that we are powerless over.

So now that we have a somewhat simple understanding of what overthinking is, I can move on to explaining what causes us to overthink different things.

The first point, to begin with, is how our modern age makes overthinking easier to do than ever. Our lives are not how they were thousands of years ago where are fears while very real, were much more well defined then "I'm stressed over exams" back then our concerns dealt more with finding food, avoiding the warring tribe next to you, or getting the hell out of dodge, when you find yourself face to face with a lion that thinks you may make a good snack. Those are all fears that have a very simple cause and effect to them.

If a lion is chasing, you then run! If you are starving to death trying to get food. Compare that to most of the fears we carry with us today "I'm worried about not passing my exam."

Well, what the hell does that even mean, from a basic standpoint?

Regarding the exam we are scared of a letter on a piece of paper, and, yes, while we can study to improve are grade and get a better letter on a piece of paper. There is not a whole lot we can do to avoid it we cannot run away from it or "fight it so to speak are best bet is to face it if we want to get our degree or whatever our goal is. The term fight or flight is one that we have all heard before. Our fight or flight response is in short, the biological response that we have developed to use when confronted with various threats. Most threats we used to be able to either fight till we either win or die or run from until we were safe, or something got us.

Compare that to now where we cannot run from most of our threats because if we do, we will find ourselves in a worse situation then we were when we first encountered said threat. This is multiplied even more with the advent of instant communication and social media where we see all kinds of famous people living lives of luxury and are sometimes reminded that we ourselves do not live a life of luxury and that our own lives do not compare. Another of the more causative factors of overthinking is putting too much stress on ourselves.

Most people like to try and achieve many different goals and to achieve goals understand that a lot of work has to be put in to meet those goals.

But it can be difficult to know where to draw the line between simply working hard toward a goal and then working yourself to death.

This is where overthinking can begin to become a negative habit. Think of it like this you begin your day by going to work spending your whole thought process towards trying to get that raise or promotion. Then you get home and what do you know your mind is still racing about it, you find yourself staring at the ceiling wondering what is going to happen if you are going to attain that goal that you want to get or if it simply going to fall flat and not become anything. Then you get up and do the same thing again.

Over a period of time, this kind of behavior can start to become quite cyclical in that you will continue to do it over and over again. In short, your brain gets used to that mode of thinking and as a result struggles with the concept that perhaps it should turn and stop running around in a circular pace. This is how overthinking truly takes root. It becomes a conditioned habit, you begin to get to the point where it becomes all you know, and you get comfortable with it. Once you become comfortable with something and it takes root as a habit it can be very difficult to break said habit. But forming a habit is much easier than it is to break a habit. Because overthinking is so heavily rooted in our mental habits it can seem easy to break because it often comes about without us even realizing it. The most important thing you can do to avoid forming a habit of overthinking is to try and cut it off right before it can take form.

This may seem challenging but realizing that things like overthinking are simply negative habits that have become ingrained is an important tool to realize. Besides becoming a reinforced habit, the other common cause of overthinking is that of stress. When we are stressed out our body releases many different chemicals like adrenaline and cortisol. These chemicals are designed to help us in a conflict such as the aforementioned lion chasing us. But they are not meant to be flowing through our veins constantly. When these chemicals are released our brain will actively try and search for a threat but it oftentimes ends up backfiring and we start to view that threat as ourselves.

Keeping stress low or to a bare minimum can allow you to actually use stress as motivation a low level of stress and anxiety can actually be optimal for getting you to complete something and get a challenging task done.

But when those chemicals start flowing too much, we then begin to find ourselves constantly overthinking and worrying about stuff. This is where overthinking really can be traced back to its root cause simply put if you are trying to get a raise or perhaps woo a girl or something. Then yes, a little bit of stress might push you forward but overexertion of said stress will simply push you back.

Avoiding stress can seem very difficult to do in this fast-paced world but the most important thing to perhaps remember is that if something is not going to actively kill you. Then worrying about it may not be in your best interest. This does not mean disregard responsibilities because they are uncomfortable or cause you a little bit of stress.

But realize that most things in this life are truly fatal, and even the things that are fatal -- well so be it, you're dead! Once you are dead you can't worry at that point! The biggest reason we like to worry is to try and feel in control about situations that seem very hard to accept. Well if you simply surrender in a sense and realize that it will be what it will be then you can avoid worrying about something that perhaps is not important.

One of the last things that can cause a lot of overthinking and also cause stress which in turn feeds into overthinking is lack of sleep. If you do not sleep well then, your brain can't take a much-needed break and will still be running when you woke up.

On top of not allowing you to rest, lack of sleep also allows stress hormones to stay at an elevated level because your body is trying to compensate for the lack of energy from not sleeping. In short, keep your stress low, your sleep good, and your habits good and you can avoid a lot of the pitfalls of overthinking.

Chapter 2: Combating Overthinking

Now that you have an understanding of what overthinking stems from and how it can affect you. I would like to now discuss how you can combat overthinking by both preventing it.

You can also stop it from becoming a bad habit.

As behaviors like overthinking are simply bad habits that get rooted within us and become hard to break. The first step in avoiding overthinking is to perhaps destroy it at the root.

The root cause for a lot of overthinking tends to come about from too much stress. Stress can come from many different places in our fast-paced modern world. As a result, identifying areas in your life that cause stress, and can actually be removed from your life can be difficult. But perhaps the most common cause for most stress in life is over employment or their personal life.

Stress over employment can seem to be unavoidable but the fact is worrying about your job constantly is not going to get you a promotion or something you need.

While stressing over your personal life or how you seem to people will not make you seem any more endearing to them. It will actually accomplish the opposite as people are good at detecting if you are stressed and nervous.

So how can you go about reducing your stress in day to day life?

Well, a change of how you look at things is one of the first steps you will want to take. What I mean by this is look at everything in the grand scheme of things.

If you are stressed out and overthinking a date you may be going on with a member of the opposite sex. Realize first that most of the fears you have inside your head are just that fears. They are not in fact grounded in reality, they are in fact grounded in unrealistic expectations that you have set for yourself or others have set for you.

While you should also realize that most of your fears are in fact false. Remember though this does not mean that every fear is false if you feel that someone seems bad or sketchy or even a situation then yes perhaps you may want to avoid it. It is great to take into account that even heaven forbid if your fears come to fruition that more often than not it is never as bad as you built it up in your head. It can be hard to change how you view stress and view your fears but the first step to take in changing your relationship to your thoughts is to practice what called grounding exercises whenever you feel yourself is getting nervous.

Grounding exercises are little mental tricks that are designed to help bring your thought processes back to a more realistic realm and help calm you down as a result of this. The most common of these is to try and look for five things you can look at five things you touch, and finally five things you can smell when you feel yourself getting stressed. This may sound stupid but what it is doing is changing the tract of your mind. You are going from worrying about whatever it is that is bothering you to now focusing on something else.

This method of changing your focus is one of the most effective tricks you can take to diminish worry and anxiety. The next step that is very important to take in your goal of diminishing overthinking is to make sure that you are getting enough sleep.

See the amount of sleep you get is heavily correlated to how well your mental health is. If you do not get an adequate amount of sleep then simply put your brain can not function as well as it should be thus making you more stressed. Now the issue here is that one of the most common causes of poor sleep hygiene is stress.

So how do you break free from this cycle?

Well, one of the best things you can do is to try and find a good routine that helps you stay calm and relaxed before you get to sleep such as taking a warm bath, reading a book, or playing a game that you enjoy.

By allowing yourself to calm down before you get ready to go to sleep, you help increase the chances of you getting a good night's sleep.

Now if you try to get better sleep hygiene and find that you are still struggling to get a decent amount of sleep then perhaps you may want to try some over the counter sleep supplements to get your sleep cycle back on track. The sleep cycle or the circadian rhythm is the internal clock all of us have that simply dictates when we get tired and when we wake up. If you have poor sleep hygiene and do not get to sleep until very late and then end uprising in the morning very late.

Well, more often than not your sleep cycle may be a bit off. The two best over the counter supplements for sleep are melatonin, a natural hormone that your own body actually produces too make you sleepy and then finally: Benadryl. Yes Benadryl, the allergy medication, when taken in a slightly higher dose (two tablets) as opposed to one act as a highly effective sleep aid.

It is best to not use this kind of medications long term but they can prove very invaluable in allowing you to get a healthier sleep cycle.

A lesser-known method for reducing stress that most people tend to ignore is actually diet.

A lot of the chemicals that are responsible for keeping us happy are actually created by the healthy bacteria that live in our stomach. This is why if you have an unhealthy diet you may actually be at a higher risk of overthinking.

So how can you combat overthinking based on diet?

Well, the first thing to understand is what exactly constitutes a poor diet. In most cases, unhealthy food can be easily defined as food that is heavily processed high in sugars and high in salt. The reason that this food can cause stress is that because it is so high in acids and bases it ends up destroying a lot of the good bacteria that is able to generate chemicals that make us happy.

The way around this is to try and stick with more natural foods, such as whole grains and organic vegetables. Thankfully if you are unable to get access to good food than one of the things that we have in our modern age are probiotics. Probiotics are simply ground up bacteria thrown into a capsule that you can take as a daily supplement.

By taking these supplements you are able to in a way cheat your own biology and allow your body to help generate these feel-good hormones without a whole lot of effort on your part. One important thing to remember is that most of these methods for reducing stress will now always take effect instantly these kinds of things take time to become normal habits and as a result do not expect them to work right away. Do not let this sound like a discouraging thing thought as by trying these things in a wide variety of ways then you will find that your mood and emotions will begin to change allowing you to make even better habits and changes in your life to allow you to reduce stress. In this world, stress can seem too hard to avoid but with the right attitude and a good mindset then yes you will be able to avoid a lot of stress and thus avoid many of the pitfalls of overthinking. And thus, you can find yourself in a much healthier mindset.

Now while overthinking is one of the more common things we can encounter in today's fast-paced society. One of the things a lot of people forget about is that overthinking is simply a form of information overload.

Think of it like this when you are thinking about something in a normal way. You are only allowing in a few thoughts at a time you are only thinking about a few important things.

When you overthink, what ends up happening is that your brain ends up filling itself with so many different thoughts. This ends up becoming what is called information overload. Think of information overload as a torrent of thoughts that fills your mind.

So, while we often go through our day to day life may be retaining a few of the things that are important to keep them with us. When we overthink, we end up holding onto everything in our head.

As a result, we allow our minds to end up being filled with a lot of things that are not required. This is a sense is what overthinking is. Thoughts fill in where they perhaps should not fill in. As a result, we end up overthinking. So how can you eliminate information overload when it comes to causing overthinking it.

Well, it can seem very difficult to control our thoughts and allow them to be somewhat simple. But the truth is that there are a couple of tactics that you as a person can take to ensure that you do not fall victim to information overload.

One of the best things you can try and do is be somewhat selective with what you allow yourself to be exposed to.

For example, instead of always checking your phone for say texts from either your boss or a lover. Sometimes it is best to simply unplug from things instead of always focusing on them. This may seem very hard in our always-on age.

But perhaps the best way to do this and also avoid information overload is to set a time range where you will not allow yourself to be constantly barraged by things. Perhaps try a 5-minute meditation 3 hours before you get home to calm your mind.

The largest cause of information overload and overthinking is simply doing too much, juggling too many activities, and trying to keep them straight in your mind is a sure way to overload your mind and get stressed out.

This is not to say that you should not put forth a lot of effort towards what you are doing but in fact quite the opposite. You need to be very selective with what you do instead of trying to do thirty things at a subpar level. Try doing less with harder effort what ends up happening when you do this is that your quality level goes up. While you also able to stay somewhat calm. This two-pronged approach is the best way to avoid information overload.

Now for some of us, information overload can come from other forms such as watching a lot of TV specifically news and always trying to focus on what is going on in our crazy world. A Lot of people focus so much on the world that they lose sight of the fact that as an individual there is not always a lot that you can do to counter things. In a sense feeling too carefully with regard to the world opens you up to a lot of hurt. As focusing on a wide variety of things that do not directly affect you as a person can put you in a position where you end up worrying about issues that may perhaps not truly matter to you. If you look at overthinking and anxiety as an irrational fear of things.

Then it becomes easier to know what kind of things you should perhaps avoid. When you are being constantly barraged with mental stimuli it can become quite easy to lose sight of what you should actually be focusing on. So perhaps instead of always spending time watching the news, or checking your work schedule with a compulsive mindset, take a step back and ask yourself how much of what you're doing at that moment will affect what you're doing.

Often worrying about something does not change the outcome and can, in fact, set you up for failure more easily the actually just relaxing and letting things pass. It can be hard to change this relationship with how you view things but if you are able to realize that most overthinking comes from a place where too much in too short of a time is hitting you then, as a result, you can easily discern what does not actually matter and what does.

Finally, for some these tactics of simply checking out to an extent do not always work. And in these situations, it may perhaps be better to try and relax throat tactics like meditation for grounding exercises. This is simply because some people are more prone to overthinking than others.

These types of people are way more likely to become flooded with all kinds of different information that really does not matter to them. This becomes the aptly named information overload where a thousand different thoughts are flooding your head instead of a few important thoughts. As when we are overloaded with too much information, we can also end up losing quite a lot of sleep which is quite bad if we are trying to stay in a calm mindset.

We find ourselves spending more time reading and researching things then we should actually sleep.

Many different things can make this easy in our modern age from stuff like social media to the 24-hour news cycle. But remember if something does not actually have an effect or influence on your life outside of hype or fear then maybe you should ignore it and pay more attention to what does matter.

Finally, try and be selective with the kind of information you allow yourself to think about instead of trying to do a hundred things at once, you will find yourself much calmer if you do this. As too much information ends up clouding your judgment and making it very hard to do what is important in your life.

Knowing how to declutter your mind is perhaps one of the best methods one can use to avoid information overload and thus prevent overthinking.

As I wrote earlier in a simple way overthinking is perhaps best described as what is called information overload gone rampant. We end up filling our minds with a wide variety of thoughts and things that have no real bearing on us as humans and as a result, end up spending time thinking about these things. This then leads to overthinking we start to lose the ability to be selective with what we think about and how we think.

See, some things do deserve a large amount of mental energy but when it gets to the point where we are thinking constantly about either our job, our relationship or even how we are spending our time.

We end up reaching a point where we lose sight of what actually matters. This is where decluttering your mind comes into play. Once you can realize what is worth your time and what is not worth you are paying attention to. You can then figure out what to keep with you and what to remove.

There are a couple of effective ways to declutter your mind that you can practice pretty much anywhere.

These are things such as meditation, calming exercises, and grounding. I would like to begin by giving a brief description of the first which is meditation. Most of us have heard of meditation and how it relates to certain religious figures like the Dalai Lama or various monks.

But did you ever stop to think that this kind of meditative practices can be applied to your life regardless of who or even where you are? There are a couple of different forms of meditation that are good for staying calm. Mindfulness meditation is perhaps the most effective for decluttering your mind. Mindfulness meditation is designed to allow you to live more presently in the moment as opposed to always thinking about either the past or future.

Mindfulness meditation can be practiced quite easily the most efficient way to practice it is to first begin by breathing in slowly for a hold of three and breathing out for a hold of three. This helps calm you down and declutter your mind in two ways the first way is that it helps lower your level of stress hormones.

The second way is that it gets you to focus on breathing instead of what is going on in your head. This can be practiced whenever you want to and whenever you need to.

Another thing to remember about decluttering your mind is that sometimes distracting yourself is the best way to do it. What I mean by this is you will want to perhaps read a book or do something that you find calming as opposed to always trying to let your mind wander. As when you find something you can distract yourself with you end up getting into a position where your brain ends up forgetting the things you were worrying about as a result you can find yourself in a very calm state of being.

Feeding into the same idea of distracting yourself another great way to declutter your mind actually involves tricking your mind. The way this will work is simply put you will trick yourself into thinking you have completed tasks that make you overthink. One of the best ways of achieving this is by making a task list of what you are going to do and from there slowly knocking off each task throughout the day.

This may seem like a relatively obvious way of completing tasks and doing work. But it plays on a very simple psychological principle and that is the fact that we as humans like to complete tasks. So, by making it to where you can check off things you have completed you in a sense can find yourself feeling even better about things you have finished as a result you may find that you are not worrying as much about various things that are going on in your life.

Now changing how you view things in your mind and begin to view them as more object-oriented and less about you also allows for easy decluttering. As you have now changed how you view your anxiety and overthinking it is now easier to fix it.

If you always assume something is about you it becomes quite easy to get worked up over nothing because you're going always assume you are going to be in a position of victimization.

When you change how you view the task or thing you are worrying about it can become much easier for you to accept things as they are. Moving backward a bit to the subject of meditation one of the great things that you can do in conjunction with meditation is allow yourself a time in which you have designated to unwind. This is perhaps the most effective way to declutter yourself.

By combining these two things you allow yourself to very quickly become calm as opposed to worrying. The first reason that this method works so well is that it begins to act as a positive habit and as a result, you can start changing your mental thought habits. What I mean by this is that the more often you can have a calm and uncluttered mind. The more often your mind will stay calm the more often you end up being calm.

This is because quite a bit of how you think is habitual. This goes the same way for having a cluttered mind. If you are always stressing out over something and filling your head with pointless things, then you are more likely to keep doing that. The other factor that meditation plays into is how it becomes easier the more you do it.

Meditation is a skill like any other and as a result of this, it takes a little bit of time to slowly get better at it. This may sound discouraging but in fact it is actually quite a good thing. Because the more you practice this kind of decluttering tricks the better you get at them and the more calm you will slowly become.

Over time this can lead to you getting better at both to such a degree that you may not need to always use them. Mental decluttering may seem like a daunting task at first but the more you practice these various techniques the more effective they become. It is important to remember to start slow with things like this instead of trying to jump in and do them at an extremely high level.

Remember to not let this discourage you as you may not see instant results instead things may take a while before they become actually noticeable and infants start to improve your life. With this attitude in mind it can become in fact quite easy to actually overcome anxiety and to a larger degree get over the plague that is overthinking. Between changing how you view overthinking and how you deal with it in no time you can quickly conquer it.

Now while defeating overthinking and information overload can seem somewhat easy at first. There are quite a few issues that can arise if you let these things fester. Just like an infected wound if these things are not treated in the beginning, they will only get worse and continue to infect your mind.

By having all of these unimportant thoughts in your mind and letting them continue to build. It can become quite difficult to discern what is important from what is not important.

Let's begin by first taking a look at what having a cluttered mind means. In simple terms, imagine if you say only have around three thousand thoughts a day and most of those are about things that matter. Such as when you are going to go to work or when you're going to make dinner. If your mind is cluttered that 3 thousand thoughts can quickly become thirty thousand. This is obviously not good because you end up losing sight of what is important.

So how does this manifest itself. Well, it can manifest in a wide variety of ways. The first way I mentioned is how it makes it difficult for you to discern what you should be focusing on. As opposed to what actually doesn't matter. But one of the more intrusive ways that always having a cluttered mind can cause harm to you is by increasing your level of stress.

Think of it like this: if your mind is always racing and always filled with pointless stuff, and you then begin to always start worrying about stuff, then at a certain point your mind becomes unable to know that perhaps worrying about stuff is possibly not the best approach to things.

So, as a result, you end up being more worried than you began with. A lot of stress can come more stress. It will begin to become difficult to get to sleep hard to actually relax. Well, when a lack of sleep is mixed with a large amount of stress that the level of stress will continue to build up. In a lot of ways stress and overthinking is a never-ending cycle. This is why it is of the utmost importance to try and break that cycle as soon as you can as opposed to always letting it sit and fester and continue.

An often-overlooked way in which having all these unimportant thoughts can harm you is how it may begin to affect your relationships.

If you are always stressed and always worried about what may come next. You end up neglecting what is going on around you and what is going on around you can often times include loved ones.

Think of it like this if you are always stressed overwork and are having a hard time leaving your work behind you when you go home then you can end up inadvertently treating loved one's kind of poorly.

This is where the most dangerous aspect of overthinking plays into because if your loved ones start getting rightly angry at how you are treating them due to you being stressed overwork. Then this stress begins to build even more as a result of you having to deal with the new added stress of your family being irritated with you. This is why overthinking and having a clouded mind can be so dangerous you end up losing sight of what truly matters. And that is perhaps more harmful than any anxiety you could ever have over something. If you're in a position where you do not know where or what is important in your life it becomes very easy for a lot of bad things to happen to you very quickly.

This is why it is very important to try and de-stress when you are at home and avoid overthinking and stress as much as you can.

While having a cluttered mind can obviously lead to a degradation of your interpersonal relationships one thing a lot of people also forget is that by being stressed and having your mind race all the time you can end up reaching a place where you begin to actually forget who you are to a degree.

While also beginning to lose sight of what actually matters to you as a person. This becomes easier the more junk you have filled up in your brain. While also causing a lot of stress in your personal life constantly overthinking and stressed can make it very hard to go and make normal decisions about seemingly basic things.

You can get to a point where even things such as simply trying to decide what you want to eat can seem like an insurmountable task. This is because you have reached the point where you are constantly trying to decide something but instead of making a decision your mind is just racing back and forth and as a result, you can't make clean decisions.

Because at that point that style of thinking has now become a habit and a habit that can be very difficult to break. This is why breaking the cycle of overthinking as soon as possible is very important to try and do. If you feel as though you cannot break the habit right away, then your best bet is to try and at least begin trying to develop healthy habits with the end goal being breaking these habits and getting to the point where you can think more freely.

Even if you cannot do these things then you can at least get to a point where you can start to change things instead of letting them constantly stay the same. Even a small change will begin to allow some positive changes to how you think.

Thus, getting you on track toward improving your mind and beginning to declutter yourself from overthinking. In doing this you allow yourself to be set up for more effective and better changes. If you don't begin to do the things required to start making these positive changes then this method of thinking is going to end up staying with you for a while and will end up harming you in the wrong one.

Chapter 3: The Power of Your Mind

As I said earlier, most of how we think is habitual in that we develop a certain style of thinking that can often carry over into how we behave throughout our day to day activities. This is why we end up with negative thinking styles as people.

Because we end up falling into bad habits such as missing sleep or drinking too much. Which end up generating more stress then they should actually help remove. This feeds into a negative cycle which leaves us more and more inclined to have bad thoughts. This is why trying to develop productive habits is so important. If you can start thinking and behaving in a manner that benefits you. You will end up better off in the end.

This is why trying to develop healthy habits is so important. If you can begin to develop a healthy way of thinking, then you can slowly come to find a way of being in which.

You can avoid this kind of negativity all together. This can be challenging at first as breaking a habit is much more difficult than it is to actually establish a habit. But on average it takes about twenty-eight days to create a habit.

One of the more common negative habits people have today is not getting enough sleep or getting to sleep too late. This can be quite a destructive habit as it places you into a cycle of always being tired and then always trying to compensate for how tired you are by other drinking coffee or doing whatever you do to stay awake.

Thus, when you need to go to sleep the following night you may end up finding yourself struggling to get a good night's sleep. Habits like these are the most common along with things like overeating, drinking too much or smoking. They are all things that at the moment make us feel good or help put off an unpleasant feeling. But in the end, they end up leaving us worse off than we were before we began them.

The best way to break a habit like this is to first understand what it is you are trying to change. Figure out exactly what habit you want to break and why. If you want to quit smoking, for example, right a list of why you want to quit and why you think you should quit. This helps get you more motivated to make a change because instead of it seeming like something super nebulous as "quit smoking" you have gone about and put it in simpler terms for you to understand and comprehend. This makes it so you can build a concrete plan toward achieving your goal.

The next step from here after having laid out the habit you want to break. Is to begin by taking slow steps towards changing your habits. Doing this slowly allows you to take baby steps toward completing your goal which allows for the goal to seem less daunting in the first place.

Now while you can break bad habits through doing stuff like this it can sometimes be in your best interest to avoid letting these habits becoming habits in the first place. Some things can become habits without us even knowing. Take for example constantly overthinking. It doesn't tend to become an issue until it starts to interfere with your day to day life. But the problem is that by the time we recognize something is starting to negatively affect us it has most likely already became an ingrained habit in our mind and as a result, we may have a hard time going about pretending.

So, the first thing you may want to do is from time to time take a bit of a personal inventory of your behavior and how you act. Doing this allows you to be on the lookout for any potential pitfalls you may encounter. This may sound like something that seems pointless.

But if you do not know how you behave and how you act then how can you go about changing yourself in the first place. The second more critical part of avoiding bad habits is to try and make sure you are not surrounding yourself with negative influences that make you more likely to form said bad habits in the first place. What this means is if you are with people who are always negative and always worrying about something and dumping all their emotions on you. It may be best to try and cut them out of your life and go about trying to distance yourself from them. As their negative behavior after a while will begin to influence your own behavior. As a result of this, you may slowly find yourself gaining some of the behaviors that they have that you do not like.

Now good habits are much harder to come across then bad habits things like getting to sleep early not smoking or drinking to excess and having time to yourself to relax. These are all examples of good habits.

The problem is that cultivating this kind of habits is much more challenging at first then cultivating bad habits. That is because sometimes what is perhaps best for us may not actually be the most comfortable thing for us to go about doing. Take working out for example at first it is a slog to try and get in reps for whatever exercise you are trying to do. You may also feel physically worse in the earlier stages of adapting to a new workout routine. But over time you will actually begin to feel a lot better than compared to when you started. As your body and mind have reached a point where they are now used to the extra physical stress and can now benefit from it.

The same goes for any good habit. Practicing things like mindfulness meditation or anything really that calms you down long term. It can seem like such a slog. But if you do not practice these things you end up setting yourself up for failure later down the road. What will most likely end up happening is that your bad habits will become further ingrained in your head and you will continue to practice them with a degree of ignorance.

Some of the simplest good habits to begin taking up are actually the simple things like having a good diet and getting to sleep at a decent hour.

The reason things like this are so important are they help us to maintain good habits all around.

Good health is crucial to our day to day functioning and life. If you have a poor diet and are not getting the nutrition that you require to operate healthily during the day. Then it won't be surprised when you begin to act in a sour mood as a result. The same can be said for when you are trying to get some sleep and end up getting to bed super late hour. This ends up making you feel rough.

Now that you have a bit of an understanding as to why both good and bad habits are an important thing to be aware of, I would like to move on and discuss how you can more effectively remove negative influences from your life.

Most bad habits tend to come about as a result of the influences around us. Say for example you work a high-stress job and are always getting home late and as a result, are always in a bad mood when you come home. Then, in that case, your place of work is influencing you to form bad habits to a degree. The same can be said if you have a friend who is always being negative. After a while, that constant spiral of negativity and stress will rub off on you.

The odd thing about negative influences is that the way they affect us tends to be in a more subtle way. Simply put by the time that we realize something is influencing us negatively the damage from it has already been done. A large amount of the media we are always consuming on either are smart devices or TV's doesn't help either.

Think back to the last time you turned on the news was the story they were reporting on something that was positive. Or was it something that was depressing and negative. Often time the answer is the latter. We can easily lose sight of this after a while and begin to think that the horror stories we hear on the news are the everyday norm. But in fact, that is not quite true the media does a very good job of trying to suck us in and get us invested into what they are selling. Tragedy sells well.

Now, to avoid stuff like depressing news we can simply just turn off the television and ignore what is going on.

That's pretty damn easy to do.

But when it comes to friends or family who are a negative influence on us it can seem like a very difficult challenge to try and remove their negative influence from us. Take for example having a friend who is a drunkard. In the beginning it can be very fun to hang out with them and go and party all the time. But after a while, their behavior can sometimes begin to drag you down. Even though you enjoy their company you can begin to reach a point where you feel like they may not be the best for you. This is where it can get difficult.

With people who are close to you in life, you end up facing the challenging question of whether their company is worth it to you. Or if you being the best person you can be at that moment is the most important thing.

So how exactly do toxic people go about negatively influencing you?

Well, the first thing that tends to happen is you begin to pick up a lot of their behaviors over time. These behaviors when they begin to show themselves can seem like perhaps your friend is just in a bad mood or is perhaps not even meaning something bad. But over time what will end up happening is you will find yourself sucked into their little whirlwind of negativity to such a degree that you begin to lose sight of yourself.

This is where you should decide how and if you want to break off from negative people. The first thing to consider is how they may act. A Lot of negative people tend to respond poorly when you bring up the fact that they are actually negative individuals so as a result of this you may want to tread somewhat carefully around them with the end goal being that you can defuse the situation. The simplest way you can do this is by slowly cutting them out of your life once you realize how their behavior is affecting you. So, start by slowly hanging out with them less and less.

Until you get to a point where you can ignore them at all. This is better than outright confrontation since they will most likely want you to stay because they feel as if they are getting something out of your relationship with them. After you remove a negative person from your life take some time to reflect back on what about their behavior you found to be negative. This is so in the future you can avoid those kinds of people while also avoiding becoming a negative individual yourself.

Now while removing yourself from negative friends can be challenging it is not as hard as trying to disconnect from a toxic family member. We all have that family member who loves to start drama and bring everyone into their little circle of chaos. These kinds of people are perhaps the worst for us to be around for a few reasons. The first is that oftentimes other family members will simply go along and put up with their negative and toxic behavior. Thus, emboldening them and allowing them to continue with the same kind of behavior we dislike.

The other reason dealing with these types of people can be so challenging is that we oftentimes find yourself thinking that perhaps we should give them a pass because they are family. But this idea that we should let them get away with their bad behavior is a further symptom of overthinking.

We are putting their poor behavior and well-being before ours. Think of it in terms of a toxic relationship. If someone is always treating you poorly and acting abusive then you would not put up with them and would perhaps leave. The same kind of mindset should be used when it comes to family members who have a negative influence on us.

What ends up happening in most of these kinds of situations is that over time we can end up spending more time dealing with their petty little issues and less time actually trying to do things in our own life. So, this begs the question of what is the best way to go about removing a family member who has a negative influence over your life.

As I said earlier, removing a family member from your life can be much more challenging to do than cutting off a toxic friend. For family is something that quite a few people hold deer regardless of the consequences that doing so might reap on them. Often times if you cut out one family member from your life you can end up inadvertently cutting of multiple family members from your life instead of just that one toxic individual. With that in mind, you will want to first ensure that you are a hundred percent serious about trying to cut out this person from your life.

Second, perhaps run by why your cutting off this person past a few family members who you know may be on your side to get an idea of how they would approach a similar situation. Finally, ensure that you keep your boundaries firm and explain to the person that you are cutting them out because you find that their behavior is having a negative impact on your life. It may be emotionally painful to do something like this at first but in the long term you are better off for doing it. The negative influence someone who is supposedly family can have on you is oftentimes greater than that of a random individual.

They can become quite good at sucking you into their own problems thus making you overthink things that would normally have no bearing on your life. Often times it is the ones we love the most who can end up sometimes hurting us. Another point to realize is that is much easier to overthink things with regards to family because of our emotions toward them. We tend to be more willing to put up with things that perhaps we would not let other people do.

Overthinking stressful things regarding family will only make anxiety and worse. While it may be painful to cut someone off like an infected limb it sometimes may be necessary for us to do for our own well-being. Negative influences are all around us in this high paced modern world.

The important thing is knowing how to avoid them and defuse any issues they may bring us. In doing this we can end up being a much calmer and more level-headed person then we have ever been before. While if we continue to let negative influences impact us then we can become stressed and spiteful person thus furthering are issues and becoming a perpetual cycle. Knowing the cyclical nature of overthinking and how external issues can influence us, especially those that are negative and also those that are caused by people. Allows us to better prepare for dealing with these types of things in the future.

After introducing how habits both good and bad can affect us. As well as how they can other set us up for great failure or great success. I would like to discuss how you as an individual can go about forming good habits and how to reap the most from the introduction of these kind of things in your life.

We all know that too much of a good thing can be extremely bad for us whether that be drinking too much, sleeping in late or worrying constantly. It can often seem hard to figure out what is good for us and what is bad.

Often times as a result of this mental disconnect we can lose sight of how simple it can be to improve our lives. While removing bad habits from our life is only a small portion of the fight towards improving yourself. If we do not replace those behaviors with positive habits, then in more ways than one there is perhaps no point in trying to improve our behavior in the first place.

The good news is that the habits that influence our behavior most often times the easiest habits for us to change. They are the things we already do day to day such as sleeping right, eating well, and maintaining a low level of stress.

Overthinking is often rooted in a series of poor habits that we can easily change. Take for example someone who does not get enough sleep well if you are tired all the time then you are going to be more prone to stress and overthinking due to the fact that you are starting your day off already stressed from said lack of sleep. These things can end up compounding on each other all with the effect of making us overthink and stress more which then leads to us reaching a crazy point where we begin to stress out over stressing out.

Even if we remove the bad habits that are causing us to overthink all the time and make us stressed. If we do not replace them with better, healthier habits it becomes very easy to fall right back into the types of behaviors that generated those bad habits in the first place. So, to begin learning any new habit it is important to go toward it with an open mind and be willing to make some uncomfortable changes. I would like to start off by discussing one of the easiest habits you can develop. That habit is getting a good amount of sleep.

Most people tend to be under the assumption that the way we sleep is somewhat of a random thing that we do not have a whole lot of control over. Well, in fact, the opposite is true the way we get to sleep is often decided by our own internal biological clock. This clock helps to tell our brain when to release chemicals to make us sleepy, and when to release chemicals to make us awake.

Think back to a time where you may be spent a lot of time on the computer or in front of any kind of screen for hours on end. You may have noticed that when you tried to get to sleep that night that you found it harder to fall asleep than normal and then woke up all groggy and irritated. That is due to you throwing off that little internal clock. Fixing your sleep schedule so you get both an adequate amount of sleep and a deep sleep is not too challenging of a task, it will require a bit of patience and dedication to see it all the way through. Because even though you can begin trying to sleep better you will not notice the results instantly.

To begin trying to repair your sleep. You're going to want to first try and keep track of how well you already sleep before you begin this. This can be done by simply writing down what time went to sleep that night. And then upon waking writing how well you thought you slept and what time you woke up.

By doing this you make it easier to know where you should improve upon and what area needs the most improvement. Once you are able to figure out if you sleep well or not you can begin the next step. An important thing to realize about sleep is that it can easily be interrupted by things like stress or unneeded anxiety. Often times people like to watch TV or play a computer game before they go to sleep.

In theory, this sounds like it should work because you are doing something that you enjoy. But in practice, anything that keeps your mind stimulated and running is going to end up being very counterintuitive toward your goal of getting sleep.

Developing a ritual of sorts before you go to sleep is the best way to ensure that you can get a consistent amount of sleep every night. This means try and do the same tasks around the same time every time you are going to fall asleep this helps trick your mind into getting ready for bed. Say you plan on going to sleep at 11:30 and it is currently ten o clock you are going to want to start getting ready for bed at ten.

Do what you normally do brush your teeth take a shower, eat, etc. Then by the time you are ready for sleep instead of watching TV or using a computer try to do something more calming like listening to a white noise machine or reading a book.

Simply put anything you can do that will relax you in the hour or two before sleep is going to help ensure that you sleep better that night.

This will not have immediate improvement in your sleep. But if you can consistently do these things every night before bed then what you will come to find is that you get both more sleep and a higher quality of sleep then you had obtained before.

Most importantly you will begin to notice that you are less stressed throughout the day and are perhaps even happier. This is due to the fact that sleep and sleep quality is heavily connected to your mental health. If you do not get enough sleep and are constantly stressed, then when you actually want to get some rest it is going to be more difficult than usual due to the fact that you have all that pent-up energy.

An often-overlooked method that you can use to help get your sleep back on track is the use of some over the counter sleep aids. Most importantly melatonin, melatonin is a hormone are brains produce at night to help make us sleepy. This chemical is released once it starts to get dark out. While when we are exposed to bright lights such as computer or phone screens are brain will stop releasing it. This is why avoiding screen time before sleep is so critical.

As a result of melatonin being produced naturally from our brain, we can safely take it as a supplement to help get us back in a normal rhythm of sleep. While sleep is an important part of a well-rounded lifestyle.

Another often missed facet that is responsible for our mental wellbeing is how well we eat. A lot of the chemicals that are responsible for making us happy are produced in our gut by good bacteria. As a result of a lot of the overproduced food we have these good bacteria can be killed. As a result of this these good bacteria end up dying. These bacteria while also being responsible for the production of chemicals that make us happy. Also help regulate sleep. While there are some bacteria that produce chemicals that make us happy.

Another often overlooked component of diet is vitamin deficiency. When you are spending a lot of your time eating foods that are heavily salted and extremely processed you can miss out on some important vitamins such as D, K, and A. These vitamins help is body produces various feel-good chemicals and without them, we can become more prone to overthinking.

The good news is that while it may seem very hard to avoid over-processed foods it is easy enough to get the vitamins that we need from other sources. To go about developing a healthy diet you are going to want to go about using the same method I described for when you are trying to improve your sleep.

Try to create a record of what kind of foods you are eating and where they are from. Once you do this you can get an idea of what kind of foods you should be cutting out. The healthiest foods are generally going to be things that are mostly natural leafy and green. Foods such as kale, salad, broccoli, and the like.

Now if you feel that you may have a hard time changing your diet you can always go about taking probiotics and vitamin tablets. But beware of this kind of things are not as effective as just changing your diet to be a healthier mix. Probiotics are simply dried bacteria that are beneficial for your gut and help your system produce these feel-good chemicals while also helping you break down various toxins in your body.

The same can be said for vitamin tables they simply introduce the missing chemicals into your body through other means. This is not a permanent fix but is one that can help you in the short term. Now while things like improving your diet and trying to get better sleep are more easily obtainable habits to develop. It is paramount to understand how to develop healthier habits in general so you can use the skills you have learned and apply them to many different facets of your life.

So how do you go about developing any habit?

Well, the first thing to keep in mind is to decide what is your end goal.

What are you trying to achieve by developing this healthy habit and how will it help you further yourself and help you achieve the things that you want to achieve?

This can be accomplished in a variety of ways but perhaps the most effective way to do this is by writing a list of what you are trying to change and how you go about doing it. See when you write something down instead of just keeping it in your head you end up making it more concrete and real to yourself.

From here you're going to want to start applying those things to what you are trying to accomplish. If you are trying to work out more frequently then make a list of the kind of exercises that you plan on doing and how many times you plan on performing them. Then begin working out but start slow and work your way up. It takes a while for something to become a habit for you generally around a month before a new behavior becomes ingrained as a habit. From here you can more easily go about obtaining your goal sense at this point it will not seem like it is some far away things that you feel as if you cannot attain.

This may seem nebulous but the truth is that any goal can be gained if you set yourself to it and doing it in a step by step method is the best way to go about getting any habit made.

Now we all know that things like eating healthy and having a good amount of sleep are all beneficial for us. But how do other habits go about benefiting us when it comes to defeating overthinking

Well, it's simpler than you may have thought. When you fill your life up with positive things such as good goals and positive influences you will quickly find that your attitude will change.

Often times anxiety and overthinking can make us feel powerless over the direction our lives are going due to how these things are able to play little tricks on our minds and get us convinced of things that perhaps are not entirely true. When this happens, we feel as though we are powerless in is goal of getting better.

So, it should make a lot of sense that when we are trying to get ourselves better than doing things that make us feel in control will make us feel as if we are in a better position in our life. If you feel in control of your life it becomes much easier to ignore those anxious thoughts.

When an anxious thought comes into your brain you are now able to almost tell it to go away. Because you now know in the back of your head you are doing everything you can to combat it. Often times we also overlook the health benefits of many healthy habits such as the ones I have mentioned so far. When you place your body in a state where it is well fed and well rested it becomes much more simple for you to be happy. Because your body now has all of the tools it needs to make you the best person you can be

Now while knowing both how good and bad habits can affect you on a superficial way is important. As well as how negative influences can increase the amount of bad habits you have. I would like to dive more in-depth into how bad habits can really increase the amount of overthinking that we do. This happens for two reasons the first is that after a certain amount of time goes by and we keep repeating the same mistakes over and over again.

We reach a point where we begin to become somewhat subconsciously aware of this fact. And as a result, when we do begin to overthink again, we can get overwhelmed by the fact that we know we are doing things that we should not be doing to a certain degree. The other facet of this problem is that most of the bad habits that people can develop.

Bad habits are things that will make us overthink and make us more anxious in the long run. As a result of this we may go back to these bad habits in the hope that we can maybe calm ourselves. And gain some clarity around what we are doing.

The most common bad habits people develop are those that are related to overconsumption. Such as drinking too much smoking too much or eating too much. Now while these kinds of habits are very common there are other more hidden habits that we can develop that can set us up for a lot of hurt. Take for instance how we react when confronted with something that makes us uncomfortable. Say you are working a job you really enjoy, and your boss calls you into the office one day and lets you know that perhaps your performance is not as good as it could be. You then get really defensive and develop somewhat of a rude tone of voice without even realizing it.

This kind of habit is more in line with our personality and as a result, can seem very difficult to change. They are very subconscious often times we do not even realize we are doing these things until we have put off a lot of people. This is why knowing how to avoid these things and break this cycle is important.

The habit of always thinking you are being attacked and someone is always trying to blame you is a dangerous one to carry with you. IT sets you up for a lot of unneeded confrontation in the sense that you will always be preparing for a fight even if there is no fight. This ties in with overthinking because oftentimes this kind of behavior result from us overthinking something and instantly assuming the worst of every situation, we are in.

This may seem like something that is easily avoidable but the truth is quite the opposite, it can be very hard to change a part of your personality but it is not impossible. The other issue with having a lot of bad habits is that they can normalize a lot of unhealthy behaviors. You reach a point where these things slowly become a part of your everyday life and you begin to think they are a normal part of being but in fact the opposite is true. You have allowed them to affect you in your day to day life to such an extent that you are now tricked into believing that.

The same goes for something that is consumption related to drinking too much. When you drink a lot to the point of being an addict it becomes quite easy to delude yourself into thinking that is normal and what everyone does. This can happen for a multitude of reasons but the two most common are as follows. Once you have begun to surround yourself with people and things that exert a negative influence upon you and as a result there is no one or nothing that can tell you to stop before things get too out of hand and to a point where this is no turning back.

So, with these points in mind on how negative habits can damage you and further increase the amount you overthink then how do you go about changing them? Well removing a bad habit is much more difficult than establishing a healthy habit. Bad habits tend to stay habits because they make us feel good and oftentimes, they are quite easy to do.

Take procrastination, for example, it is very easy to fall into a pattern where we out of something we are supposed to do because it is easier than getting to work right away. This ends up never being true and gets us into a situation where the amount of work we have to complete in a designated amount of time is more than if we had just done what we were supposed to.

This is never a good thing when looking as an observer at someone's behavior. But when you are the one doing it, it can become very difficult to realize how this behavior is damaging you.

This is what makes bad habits so dangerous we oftentimes underestimate the damage that we are doing to yourself. We oftentimes find ourselves questioning what people are saying to us and just continue doing what we are doing regardless of the consequences that it can bring upon us.

Understanding this is the hardest part of removing a bad habit. Now to actually go about changing a bad habit you need to first figure out what you are trying to change and why you want to change it. IT is much easier to change something once you realize why you are doing it.

The most effective way to do this is to make a list of what you are trying to change then just committing it to memory. Because when you leave these ideas just in your mind things can easily get changed. This is due to no fault of your own but happens as a result of the fact that the human mind loves to play tricks on itself. The other way you can prevent this from happening is to try and ask some friends to help you change whatever you're going for. Simply ask them if they can notice any noticeable change in how you act and if they are willing to help you along the way by keeping you on track. If you cannot do that then stick to writing down a list of what you are trying to change.

Now the important thing to remember about changing a habit especially if you are an individual who overthinks. Is to take it nice and slow. The reason for this is that if you try and rush and change a bunch of things at once then you can reach a point where it seems impossible to actually make any meaningful change in your life. You may end up overthinking harder than you normally do, due to the fact that you feel that you are being presented with something that you think you cannot due. The way around this is to try and quit your habit in small increments if you have a habit of blowing up at people, for example.

Begin by first recognizing what sets you off, and then from their writing up an action plan of what you are going to do when something begins to set you off and take a break from there.

Practice that step over and over again until you feel comfortable with it. By doing this you can cement these small changes and make them more permanent.

While also trying to change a bad habit takes some time to try and realize what got you to that place to begin with. If you are quitting smoking, for example, realizing why you picked up smoking in the first place allows you to realize how you can prevent going back to that old mindset in the first place. As with most things in life, practice is what makes perfect. Instead of just jumping around and trying to change things quickly and expecting that everything will be alright as a result. You ideally want to reach a point where you can gain a bit of insight into yourself by removing these bad elements from your life.

After you begin to get an idea of what habit you are trying to change. And you begin to try and change it, you may want to begin considering if you want to develop a good habit in its place.

Going back to the smoking analogy you can maybe try and replace those toxic cigarettes with healthy celery or something of the like whenever you begin to feel the urge to smoke. This allows you to trick your brain in a sense. You will no longer begin to view it as a loss and instead will view it as a win, you substitute the bad with the good.

The most important thing to remember and realize about bad habits is that if you leave and ignore them. Then they will only get worse, a bad habit, when it begins can seem pretty harmless like something you can just brush off and ignore but the opposite is in fact true. You will only find that it gets worse. This happens due to the fact that as you do something more and more and continue a behavior it becomes more ingrained in your head and becomes a more common way for you to act.

A mild drinking problem is not destructive in the beginning, but it is the prolonged damage that is the worst that is where the true issues arise when you get to the point that you believe it is the only way you can function.

This plays hand in hand with overthinking in a cyclical way.

You may try to quit a habit due to you always thinking about how bad it is for you but then you reach a point you decide one day to give up said bad habit and change things up. By the time you realize that you have an issue, and this can be an issue with anything it is already too late, in your mind. By virtue of you thinking that nothing is going to get better than habit is only going to continue to get worse and worse before it begins to eat you alive.

This is why trying to eliminate a bad habit as soon as possible is in your best interest. Also, think about it like this if you are constantly worrying about something in your life taking action is one of the best ways to ensure that you will worry left. The feeling that you are not in control of what you are doing will just continue to fester and grow as you're not going out of your way to change it.

One of the last components of breaking a bad habit that people oftentimes are reluctant to want to admit. Is that for many habits it is the people around you, who can enable you to continue these things. Often times this is simply because they are so caught up in their own mess, that do not realize the negative effects that they're having on you. It may seem like a hard truth to realize, but often you may be better off to drop these people then continue on with them.

This ties back into the subject of negative influences many of the people who we can choose to spend our time with, can influence us with their own behavior. Think about it this way if you have a friend who is always saying something bad about everyone, then it can become quite easy for you to fall into that habit yourself. This is not due to any fault of your own but, more because humans pick up on the traits of others.

Simply put, if you are always around toxicity and negativity it is not too surprising then that it may occasionally rub off on you, and thus make you toxic. Cutting people out of your life can seem like a very painful endeavor at first but the reward for not having to deal with toxic behavior is much better than allowing yourself to put up with it.

This is the kind of situation where you must weigh every option; do you value this person's friendship even if it raises the chance of damaging you? Or would you rather offend them in the hope that by cutting those out you can then begin to eliminate some toxic behavior?

Chapter 4: Meditation

Meditation is one of the best ways you can go about trying to gain a hold on overthinking.

Meditation has been practiced by people for thousands of years for a variety of different reasons, but only in recent times has it gained a resurgence here in the West for the calming benefits it can impact on people.

Simply put the idea of meditation is to clear your mind and allow yourself to relax and be calm. Meditation can come in a wide variety of forms. But the most effective one for trying to reduce mental clutter and eliminate overthinking is to try mindfulness meditation.

Practicing meditation requires little to nothing except a space where you won't be bothered. One of the greatest benefits you can gain from meditation is a permanent mindset change.

By practicing mindfulness meditation daily, you will begin to notice a steady decline in your anxiety and worries. This is because meditation helps rewire your brain to be calmer. This works well to prevent overthinking because you are working to remove the negative thought patterns that keep you trapped in a cycle of overthinking.

Meditation is perhaps one of the most efficient tools for trying to combat overthinking. See meditation allows you to break that cycle of constantly worrying and overthinking every little thing. While being an extremely effective tool for combating overthinking, meditation has the added benefit of being an all-natural practice. So, it is something that you can do alone in your own time without any required tools.

When you begin to practice meditation, you may notice that it is somewhat challenging at first. Due to how your mind will want to wander instead of simply clearing itself. The main goal of meditation is to clear your head. To focus on nothing except what is going on in the present moment. This is extremely effective for combating overthinking because it allows you to learn how to think and operate in a calmer matter.

When we overthink our mind races back and forth from point to point, in a highly convoluted mess. This obviously is not a good thing, overthinking can lead to all sorts of problems such as anxiety disorders, depression, sleep problems.

Meditation is perhaps the most powerful tool you can use to combat these ailments. As I said in the beginning of this section, meditation has been practiced for thousands of years. This is because it works, and it works well.

Meditation works to calm the body in a few different and interesting ways. Breathing as we all know is an integral part of staying alive but breathing too fast can cause us to panic. I am sure you have noticed that when some people get really worked up or stress, they may begin to hyperventilate thus making themselves panic even harder and faster. Well, this happens because when our body releases stress hormones are respiration elevates in anticipation of some external threat.

The problem is that when the threat is coming from an internal source such as our own mind, as is often the case with ailments like overthinking or just generalized anxiety. Then these mechanisms serve no purpose but to make us more panicky.

What meditation does is help slow down your breathing and allow more oxygen to travel throughout your body as opposed to carbon dioxide, which elevates our stress levels. When we are able to slow our breathing and gain a grip on what is going on, we end up focusing less on what is running back and forth in our minds and more on our breathing. This idea of breath is the central crux of meditation. If you can manage to control how you breathe and how fast your breathing you will find that you quickly reach a calm state.

While a lot of meditation is focused on your breathing the other component attached to meditation is how your mind operates.

When you practice meditation more and more you will find that you begin to become more calm overall.

This is because meditation helps to rewire your brain to be healthier.

When we overthink all the time we can easily get caught in that cycle of overthinking. Where we will worry about things that have little to no bearing on our life. This happens partially due to faulty brain wiring we end up getting into a cycle of overthinking.

Our brain gets used to constantly over-analyzing every little thing. And as a result, it becomes a habit of ours, a habit that can be very difficult to break because we get used to it.

Now, when we practice meditation what is happening is, we are clearing our mind of excess clutter. A cluttered mind is the main thing that is responsible for the symptoms of overthinking. The way in which meditation allows us to adopt new habits of thinking is what makes it such a valuable tool. It allows us to break out of these unhealthy habits and replace them with a healthier way of thinking.

It is one thing to break a bad habit. Yes, it is good to remove bad habits, but if we do not replace them with something more positive then it becomes very easy to fall back on to the same old behaviors. With meditation we end up replacing the habit of overthinking with the exact opposite, we allow ourselves to reach a state of calm. The more often we can calm ourselves the more natural it will come to us as a result.

One of the often under looked benefits of practicing meditation regularly, are the health benefits that you can infer from it as a result. See when you meditate you lower a few important body levels. See when we get stressed out things like our heart rate and blood pressure rise. This is highly harmful for our bodies as it causes undue stress on our organs.

When we can lower all of these things as a result of calming ourselves. We are not only making yourself happier, but we are also improving our health, which in turn can lead to more happiness. Now it should be said that meditating before we go to bed is perhaps the most efficient way to begin practicing meditation.

The reason for this is quite simple. When we overthink, we can often find ourselves having difficulty getting to sleep and also having a challenging time getting deep sleep.

Meditation relaxes us and makes us calm, so as a result when done before bed you help increase the chances that you will gain a restful and calming sleep. This practice of meditating before bed is a great habit to add to your nightly ritual.

Before diving too deeply into meditation I would like to step back to the earlier discussion of using meditation to further combat overthinking this time with a bit more in detail how you can use it to not only stop overthinking in its tracks but also prevent further bad habits from forming.

One of the biggest issues that happens with overthinking is the fact that it becomes habitual very, very quickly. A lot of bad habits can feed into overthinking, such as constantly thinking people are mad at you are always playing the victim.

While, yes, constantly being stressed all the time will most definitely add to your level of overthinking, having bad habits can also go about making overthinking, much worse. See when we get angry constantly or drink too much in the hopes that these things will help us be better people or calmer.

We often reach a point where we finally decide to break these bad habits. Well to break a habit is good and most definitely a helpful thing to try and conquer overthinking. If you are unable to figure out why you developed that habit in the first place, then you run the risk of falling back on that habit some time again in the future.

Through meditation, you can sometimes come to an understanding of why you do these things and how they affect you.

We know that meditation slows down our thoughts and allows us to be more clear-headed, well, as a result, you can sometimes come to realize things that you may not have normally considered. Because when you are calm as opposed to tense and angry it is much easier, to figure out why and how you do something as opposed to trying to sift through your thoughts while all irate.

This is the most understated way in which meditation allows us to combat overthinking. Simply put when putting the practice of mindfulness meditation to good use daily we begin to get a better sense of who we are and where our desires lie. This is due to the fact that it allows us to get a better look inside of ourselves clutter-free and with a new mindset. Changing your mindset even just a little bit in short little increments like you can accomplish by meditating. Makes it so that you don't have to worry about trying to improve yourself all at once. By taking a step back and looking at the whole picture instead of these little disconnected bits you gain a sense of calmness that you perhaps would not normally gain elsewhere.

Finally, one last piece of advice I would like to leave you with before finishing this section is to not be intimidated by all of the different forms of meditation that are out there. Really the only form of meditation that will really benefit you is mindfulness meditation, and this is because it is a practice that is designed to calm you and make you more mindful of your surroundings. It is also the easiest to practice requiring little to nothing to actually learn how to effectively use the techniques for it.

Actually, practicing meditation is a lot simpler than you might expect.

As a practice meditation does not require any real supplies or pre-requisite skills to begin. Why no supplies? The primary tool of meditation is breathing.

Simply put when you meditate you accomplish a few things. The first thing that occurs when you meditate is that you slow down both your heart rate and speed of respiration. By slowing down these bodily functions you allow yourself to calm down, not just mentally but also from a biological standpoint. In short, you are reducing a lot of the biological process that makes you stressed and cause you to overthink in the first place.

By slowing down these bodily functions you allow your mind to mellow out. This occurs because instead of trying to focus on what is going on in your head you begin to change your focus on to your body thus calming your mind and body at the same time. So, with that and mind how do you actually begin to practice mindfulness meditation. Well, there are a few different methods that are used for practicing mindfulness meditation the first and most commonly used method only requires two things. The first thing you need before you begin actually meditating is a place where you can be unbothered.

This is perhaps the most important requirement due to the fact that your goal with this meditative practice is to clear and empty your mind.

Well, emptying your mind can be quite challenging to do if you are in an environment where various things can interrupt you. Ideally a place where you can either sit or lay comfortably also allows meditation to be accomplished easier, this is needed for the simple fact that some forms of mindfulness training work much better in an environment where you can get nice and comfortable, in short, a place where you can let it all out and truly relax. The last requirement for meditation is more of a personal trait and that is patience. You need to be patient when beginning to meditate. As with any new skill when you first start out trying to meditate it will most likely seem very challenging at first. Thoughts will bounce around in your head back and forth and you will end up finding it quite challenging to simply just be and let your thoughts flow. As a result, if you are someone who is not patient you may find meditation to be a very challenging skill to try and work on.

Once you have found a nice spot to begin meditating, ideally somewhere where you can meditate unbothered and just relax. You're going to want to first begin by sitting upright with your hands by your abdomen. This is done to allow you to breathe more deeply and more efficiently.

Since breathwork is pretty much the crux of meditation to begin with. Once you are seated in both a correct and comfortable position you can begin.

To start off first allow your mind to race, let it run back and forth as much as it wants to. Try to not engage any of the thoughts that come into your head.

Even if an uncomfortable thought passes by your head let it just flow off of you like water under a bridge. Now while your thoughts are flowing back and forth, you're going to want to begin the breathwork component. Accomplishing this is a very simple task, simply take a very deep breath in, for around five seconds. Next, hold that same breath for another count of five, and then finally exhale for five. What you're going to want to do next is practice these breathing multiple times during your meditation practice. You want to keep up this pattern of breathing for around fifteen minutes. This is done for a few different reasons, the first of which is to actually begin to calm yourself down.

With most meditation, it will be somewhat difficult at the beginning of a session, but get easier you continue breathing deeply.

This is because your body and mind are still trying to acclimate to this different form of breathing. Normally when we breathe, we take very shallow breaths and exhale them quickly. In our day to day life when we breathe, we are focusing on just getting oxygen into our bodies, and not trying to actually breathe in an efficient and comfortable manner.

After you have practiced the breathing method a few times, you can begin to try another form of mindfulness meditation that is more designed to combat fear and anxiety. For this, you want to assume the same sitting position as you normally would legs crossed, back straight up and hands at your center.

Begin with the same deep breaths as you normally would. So in for five, hold for five, and then exhale for five seconds. But now instead of just simply focusing on your breath and letting your thoughts flow back and forth within your mind.

Try to think of your largest and biggest fears. Whatever bothers you the most in life allow it to come to the center of your mind. This may seem like a scary thing to do. Every time a fear-driven thought enters your mind simply let it pass. In short, allow the fear to enter confront it and then exhale.

This may sound like a scary or frightening thing to do. In reality, what you are doing is actually unlearning your response to your thoughts. Normally when a thought enters our mind that we might characterize as anxious or convoluted our first response is to either try and push it out, or react to it.

By simply allowing the thought in and then breathing to calm yourself. You help to retrain your brain to no longer respond to these types of thoughts with fear, instead you look at it with acceptance. Accepting that something bothers you and realizing that it will shortly pass is one of the best methods you can use to tackle overthinking and anxiety. When you try and resist something that is making you uncomfortable and push it to the back of your mind. It will only begin to grow stronger and worse. Meditation helps reverse this process by putting you in a calm state and letting you relax and destress whenever an uncomfortable thought approaches you.

The benefit of learning these meditative practices does not just come from using them to simply meditate. Some of the aspects of meditation can be applied to your day to day life. Calming breathing can be applied in a multitude of situations where you may begin to feel uncomfortable.

Breathing deeply and slowly can calm you almost instantly due to the fact that first, it slows your heart rate, which will dramatically rise when feeling either anger or stress. Secondly, this kind of meditative breathing helps to slow your respiration rate, that sounds obvious I know, but realize that when you are panicked or stress you may have a tendency to breathe very rapidly both in and out.

So, to apply these tricks in your day to day life I would like to give an example. Say you are driving your way to work, and someone cuts you off and you then end up at a red-light. This is a scenario that most people would find themselves in and most people would begin to get angry and or stressed. When you feel that first pang of anger or discomfort simply begin to breathe in and out slowly and allow your mind to race.

What will begin to happen is that you will start to ignore the fact that you're at a red light, and also begin to ignore the fact that you are even stressed out to begin with. This is how meditation can be used most effectively. After a while of applying this kind of calming techniques to your daily life.

You will begin to find that you are a lot calmer in most if not all situations you encounter. I would like to close this section with a reminder that meditation while helpful is a skill and like any skill requires constant practice to ensure that you can reap all the benefits that it has to offer you as an individual.

Now while understanding meditation is one big component of practicing it.

There are a couple of tips and tricks to practicing meditation that I would like to pass along to help further you in your goal of learning of proper meditation technique that people oftentimes forget. And that is how to maintain proper posture as to allow for breathing. See meditation is primarily focused on your breath.

As mentioned earlier when we meditate, we slow down our breathing and our heart rate which in turn leads to us feeling calm while also helping us to clear our minds. It may sound simple enough to just sit down and breath but the truth of the matter is that when practicing breathing in meditation. IF your posture is not correct then without a doubt the way that you are breathing will not be correct.

Most people beginning meditation make the mistake of trying to sit down in a crossed position, this method works at first because it allows you to learn some of the beginning steps of meditation. But once you do it more and more you will begin to notice how sitting slouched makes for a less efficient meditation session. The way around this is to try and simply sit upright when you meditate. As to allow yourself to have a better ability to let air get deep into your lungs.

Now while deep breathing is an important component of meditation. As it does actually form the basis for most meditation practices. One other important part of the meditative state is to try not to rush yourself with it.

Often times the reason people do not get the best benefits from meditation is that they try to meditate for too long, too early. What I mean by this is that when you are beginning to learn any new skill, it does not usually make sense to try and spend hours at a time doing it, this is simply because you can end up learning improper form and begin to develop habits of doing that skill in the wrong way. Well, this occurs more often with meditation do to the fact that people want to try and reap most of the calming benefits of meditation at once.

The problem with this is that sense meditations main goal is to help empty your mind, if you are focusing too much on trying to calm yourself, what ends up happening is that you begin to focus on the wrong thing as a result, this is never a good thing to have happen to you as it is counterintuitive the whole goal of meditation.

To avoid this, it is highly recommended that when you first begin to meditate that instead of spending all your time focusing on how your thinking and what you are thinking about, to instead just let your thoughts flow back and forth and be a passive observer of them. As well as doing this you should also begin to try shooting for meditating around 15 minutes at a time, instead of trying to meditate for long periods of time uninterrupted.

Simply put when you first start meditating it will be very challenging for you to try and maintain a healthy amount of calmness through this whole practice, as a result, you are much better of trying it in little chunks like this. By doing all of these things bit by bit, you will be much more prepared to move on to doing meditation more regularly as you will have gained the basic skill set required for mastery of meditation!

Chapter 5: Thinking and You

Now while practices like meditation can be highly beneficial in the goal of trying to combat overthinking. There are other methods of changing your thinking that can accomplish multiple things at once.

Using some of the innate traits that we all have as humans such as creative thinking can allow us to do some very interesting things. See generally the way people will try and combat overthinking is by trying to block out those kinds of thoughts.

While that can work in the short term in trying to defeat these issues. It is not always the best way to go about trying to improve ourselves. Due to the fact that all of us are born with an innate creativity, we can utilize creative thinking to help us overcome any problem we may encounter. After all the way we solve anything we are dealing with in life is through problem-solving skills which are is just an extension of creativity.

With creative thinking in mind, how do we go about increasing our ability to be creative?

Well, this problem has a lot to do with the main subject discussed in this book overthinking. When we overthink, it can become very difficult to change what we are thinking about and where our focus lies.

This is one of the main ways in which anxiety manifests itself.

To combat this, we need to try and develop skills that allow us to think in a more clear fashion. This is where developing creative thinking skills come in to play.

One of the most efficient ways you as an individual can try and harness the power of creative thinking. Is by engaging our brain more and trying to do more activities that challenge us mentally. See the brain is like a muscle and when you make use of a muscle it only gets bigger.

This is why trying to engage creatively is so important to our mental wellbeing. If we just let our brain sit there and do nothing then it will do just that, nothing. But when we engage in things like sudoku or puzzles we help build our brain up to be more effective in how we use it. While training using various intellectually stimulating activities can help boost your brainpower.

There is no point in doing this if you do not know how to apply these kinds of things. Think of it like this every day we have thousands of thoughts that flood through our head.

How many of those thoughts actually end up being useful and can actually make a difference in our lives, very little of what we often think can have any real sort of impact.

When I say change the way you think what I am in fact referring to is being selective with what you decide to put effort into. If you put all of your effort into your fears and anxieties then yes, you're not going to gain a whole lot as a result. But instead, if you focus on trying to improve your life day to day and put forth your whole energy toward things that matter then you will be surprised at the results this can give you.

Now while most people associate creative thinking with the arts and the like most people do not realize that creative thinking can come especially handy during our day to day life. The fact is that in today's modern world we are often faced with a wide variety of different problems that tend to have a lot of possible solutions.

By using creative thinking to our advantage, we can oftentimes come up with the best possible answer in ways we may not have considered. This is where most of the benefits of training your brain comes into play. You can reach a point where you begin to solve your life's issues in a wide variety of ways.

Think about a car for example oftentimes a car will break down and our first instinct is to go to a mechanic and try and get it fixed. But when we apply our mind and use creative thinking, we can often find workarounds for various mechanical problems in areas we may not have considered.

You may have heard the term jerry-rigging this term means a simple at-home solution to a mechanical issue using parts and items that you have easily available at your disposal. Say you have a fuel line leak and you are running out of tubing, well with creative thinking you can come to the conclusion that perhaps using something like a section of garden hose may work.

This is the kind of thinking I am talking about looking at problems with an abstract lens and trying your best to find a solution with simple what you have on hand. This same approach works great when applied to overthinking. As I said earlier it is not uncommon in today's world to be constantly worrying about something and then spend way too much time trying to fix the issue. Well when you decide to think outside of the box you often will find that the best solutions tend to be the ones you would never consider

This is because of how overthinking tricks our brain when we overthink, we begin to lose sight of what really matters to us and as a result can begin to get blindsided by the world around us as a result of how our mind is operating at that time and place.

Now while creative thinking is extremely beneficial. It can oftentimes seem like a challenging thing to actually engage yourself in their often times it seems like there are a myriad of challenges in our way when we try to overthink. But if look at overthinking less as a tool and more as a different way of solving things it can begin to become easier.

You can also begin to use creative thinking to try and combat overthinking, as stated earlier overthinking is oftentimes able to cloud our judgment. And make us pay more attention to the things that perhaps do not matter to us. Well to get around that you can oftentimes find yourself trying to think outside of the box.

The problem with trying to use this method of creative thinking, is that by forcing yourself to think what ends up happening is you are boxing yourself in more. Often times the best ideas and thoughts come from places and things where we would least expect it. So, it would make sense then, that to try and force yourself to think creatively would end up backfiring and doing the opposite of what you intended.

So, this begs the question of how do you actually begin to practice creative thinking. Inspiration, we have all read or heard stories about places and events that inspire our favorite artists and creators. But few of us perhaps actually understand what inspiration is. To be inspired by something is to be moved by it in a way that you traditionally would not consider. Say you're looking at how the grass blows in the breeze and you are an engineer working on windmills. Now at first glance, these two items seem entirely unrelated to each other by virtue of them each occupying different spaces in our mind and both serving a different purpose.

But when you allow yourself to truly take in and admire what is around you that is when you can begin to learn and understand things that perhaps you would not have considered. By looking at the grass said engineer can realize how to better make turbines. Allowing yourself to try new things and go to new places accomplishes to things with one task. First, by stepping outside of your comfort zone you can help yourself to eliminate some of the mental blocks and fears that are oftentimes a result of overthinking.

When we overthink and worry a lot, we can become fearful of stepping outside of our comfort zone. As a result of this, our world can begin to seem stale and boring as a result. This can make trying to utilize the creative elements of our mind all the more difficult. So, when we finally do make that bold step and decide to try things that we are not always comfortable with we end up engaging parts of our mind that we would not normally use. Thus, enabling us to gather inspiration from different places and events

Now while creative thinking can become especially useful for trying to combat overthinking. One of the best and time-tested methods for defeating overthinking is by replacing it with positive thinking. Simply put positive thinking is where we as individuals try and think positively about what we are doing with the goal of trying to change our mood. At times this can seem like a very challenging task, especially when we are always faced with so many different issues and fears in today's modern age. But people often forget that attitude is everything and if you have the right mindset nothing is really impossible to accomplish.

See positive thinking works as a great counter to overthinking because like you do with removing bad habits you allow yourself to replace your negative thoughts with positive ones, this leads to a feeling of calm and peace. Because while negative thoughts come and go very rapidly and can seem almost impossible to counteract, positive thoughts tend to have more power than negative thoughts. There are a few ways you can cultivate a positive mindset.

One of the benefits of trying to begin positive thinking is that it ties in quite well with the meditative practices. When we meditate, we allow ourselves to become calm and begin to look at the world from a different perspective. Often times what comes about as a result of this is a change in our attitude. We will begin to look at the world more positively instead of always trying to look at the glass half empty. This tends to occur because we have shifted our focus from our nervous and worrisome thoughts to a place that is more centered and more calm.

While meditation can help you cultivate a positive attitude and more positive thoughts. One of the other ways you can get a more positive attitude is to actually practice some of the same things that are done to try and defeat a negative habit.

Writing a list of the things you are grateful for and make you happy, allows you to change how you look at the world. See instead of always looking at everything from a negative standpoint what will begin to happen as you look throughout the world from a positive mindset, is that you will begin to become more thankful for what you have and realize that perhaps your life is not as bad as it seems.

This may seem like a challenging thing to do at first but as time goes on it will become easier and easier for you to do. Now while making a list and trying to practice gratitude helps with developing a positive mindset. What good is a positive mindset if you do not know how to apply it in your day to day life.

As I have said earlier it can be quite challenging to try and actually keep a positive train of thought. But when you try and look at the larger picture of things it begins to slowly get easier and easier as time progresses. Instead of constantly worrying about what is going on around you what begins to happen is that you develop a different attitude toward things that may normally bother you.

You can begin to see the mas ways that you can improve yourself as a human being instead of challenges that are just going to set you back. So, to apply positive thinking to your day to day life what you are going to want to do is combine it with meditative practices. So, when an anxious thought comes into your head as opposed to just letting it pass what you are going to try and do is replace it with a more positive thought. By doing this you can gain a better outlook on things. To actually properly use positive thinking to counter negative thoughts you need to also realize that sometimes a negative thought is inevitable, and it may come and will eventually pass.

What you can do is to try and do is actually distract yourself with something more positive when you feel a wave of negativity hitting you. What ends up happening when you change your focus like this is you begin to fully replace that negativity with positivity something that while seeming changeling can really benefit you in ways that you may not have expected.

See by focusing on something that is more positive when you feel negative you make it easier to cultivate a positive mindset. Because as with meditation you are able to remove the association that comes with a lot of negativity you begin to slowly de condition yourself to emotionally responding to negativity.

By replacing the way, you react to things and placing a positive mindset in the place of a negative mindset. You allow yourself to gain a bit of clarity that you perhaps would not normally have this, in turn, allows for a great change in your being and in your mind. Which is always a great thing to have happen.

While positive thinking can seem like a challenging ordeal to try and accomplish at first the most important thing to remember before embarking on trying to change your mental mindset is to keep yourself open to the types of changes that may come as a result. See at the beginning of trying to change your attitude and mental mindset you may find yourself potentially scared to a degree.

This is, in fact, a normal thing to have happen because you are beginning the process of trying to engage in a new way of living. This is always a challenging task for anyone to accomplish. See when you go into something with a closed mind which is quite common to do when you are suffering from the effects of overthinking. You become apprehensive to any new form of change. Which is to be expected as humans are somewhat adverse to change.

But change is one of the few constants in the universe.

If you can accept this fact you will be much more receptive to what is going on around you. And as a result, it will become much easier to change yourself for the better. While trying to change how your attitude functions may seem like a daunting task at first, the truth is quite the opposite. It's simpler than you think to try and change your attitude once you know the benefits that you can gain from that.

The benefits of positive thinking are oftentimes quite understated. Positive thinking simply means trying to maintain a positive attitude in the face of adversity. It does not mean as some people think trying to keep all your thoughts positive all the time.

Doing that is quite difficult to do and can prove to be very challenging. For the most part, we do not really control a lot of the thoughts that enter our heads constantly. Most of our thoughts come about as a result of external and internal stimuli, that our brain then transforms into thought.

While our attitude is more the result of how we view the things, we go through. We can decide if we let something build us up or beat us down. This is very simple for us to do because we can kind of consciously decide how we will go about tackling a problem.

Out of all the myriad of thoughts that can fill our head at any given time to a certain degree, we can pick and choose what we decide to focus on. We can choose if we wish to make a damaging choice in fixing our problems or a positive choice in trying to solve the issues that affect us from a day to day perspective. This is where some of the true benefits of trying positive thinking really begin to show. You reach a point where now that your attitude has changed you can change.

Chapter 6: Sleep and You

We all know the crummy feeling that comes with not getting enough rest at night but I don't think many people stop to ever realize how a lack of sleep can make the issues associated with overthinking both worse and make them occur more often. When we sleep our brain is given a time and also catalog memories. Sleep allows a lot of different brain chemicals to be set back to a decent level

These are the same chemicals that are responsible for causing stress responses and also giving us anxiety. When we don't sleep these chemical levels end uprising and thus causing more stress. It is easy to view sleep just as a thing we all have to do by virtue of being a human. But the fact is like anything else in your life sleep is a habit.

We all have in our body what is called a circadian rhythm this is also known as our sleep cycle. How and when we get to sleep is controlled by a wide variety of external and internal factors. One of the biggest issues with trying to get to sleep at a decent time in this modern world. is the prevalence of electronics, computer and television screens can keep us up through two methods the first is how they stimulate our brain?

If you are watching a television show chances are your mind is racing back in forth in regards to whatever it is your watching.

This ends up stimulating you in a wide variety of ways mentally, thus making your brain run back and forth quicker making it more challenging to actually get to sleep. Secondly, the light from a television or laptop screen messes with some of our most important brain functions, these are the parts of our brain that are responsible for our wake and sleep functions.

We all produce a hormone in our brain called melatonin, melatonin is responsible for telling our body when to make us tired and when to put us to sleep. Our brain stops the release of melatonin in response to exposure to light and releases it when it gets dark outside. As a result of how screens are so brightly illuminated the release of this very important chemical can end up getting inhibited and as a result, we end up staying awake. There is one very simple way thought that you can combat this.

Before going to bed and at least 45 minutes before preparing for sleep you want to try and avoid most if not all brightly illuminated screens. That can seem very hard to do with how prevalent the use of technology is in today's society. But doing this is worth the extra sleep you can get. If you want to see this in hard facts take a look at this chart that shows the correlation between screen time and poor sleep quality. The results of this will most likely surprise you.

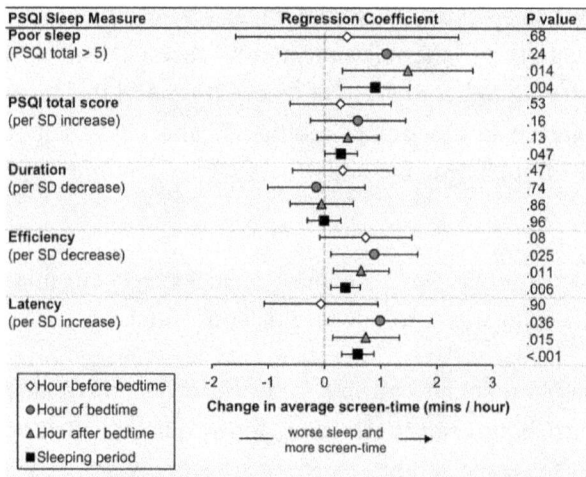

PSQI Sleep Measure	Regression Coefficient	P value
Poor sleep (PSQI total > 5)		.68
		.24
		.014
		.004
PSQI total score (per SD increase)		.53
		.16
		.13
		.047
Duration (per SD decrease)		.47
		.74
		.86
		.96
Efficiency (per SD decrease)		.08
		.025
		.011
		.006
Latency (per SD increase)		.90
		.036
		.015
		<.001

	-2 -1 0 1 2 3
◇ Hour before bedtime	Change in average screen-time (mins / hour)
● Hour of bedtime	
▲ Hour after bedtime	____ worse sleep and more screen-time →
■ Sleeping period	

Now while screens can play a big role in keeping us from getting the kind of restful sleep that we need to be a productive individual. Having

74

what is called poor sleep hygiene can also play a part in not getting enough rest.

Sleep hygiene is a fancy term for the habits and patterns that we all have that allow us to get to sleep and the environment that we sleep in. This may come as a bit of a surprise but before and during sleep your body goes through a whole host of different metabolic changes such as lowering your core temperature a few degrees, inhibiting certain reflexes and the like. Well, a lot of these things cannot happen if you are not doing the right things to allow them to happen. Take for instance temperature us humans sleep best when it is around 73 to 68 degrees Fahrenheit in the bedroom.

This is because that cold temperature helps slow down our bodies and get us more prepared for rest. Another addition and more important factor of trying to get a good night's sleep is to make sure that you can develop a healthy routine every night before you go to bed. See when we do certain things before going to bed like brushing our teeth or taking a hot bath and then promptly after going to sleep.

We begin to trick our brain into thinking that this is the time for us to go to sleep. Developing a healthy ritual before we go to sleep s so important due to the fact that it is what prompts us to start getting sleepy and calm down.

Sleep is very much a habitual and cyclical so to go about developing or changing a sleep habit can prove to be difficult but there are a few ways you can develop a sure-fire healthy sleep method. The first thing you're going to want to do is try and ensure that when you begin to get ready for bed you choose a consistent time to always do so.

So instead of say trying to get to sleep at a different time every night tries and find a set time where you can begin to get ready for bed and try and stick to it. This will allow you to get the best sleep you can. When you can begin to do this, you will find that it becomes easier the more you do it. This is very important to try and remember because at first, you may be somewhat apprehensive about trying to adapt new sleep habits into your life.

But as a result of this happening you can first be scared of trying to adopt these new sleep habits. The biggest thing that you have to lose from not getting enough sleep is that your mental health will begin to reach a cyclical state, and you will begin to find it somewhat challenging to try and get an adequate amount of rest that is required for all of us. Thus, making you more stressed and cranky upon waking and leading you to having a difficult time getting to sleep the following night.

While trying to cut out a lot of the time you spend on a screen before bed can help you get more sleep and also better sleep at that. There is also a great deal of importance on where you sleep. Most people sleep in their bedroom.

Simply because this has their bed and becomes the spot that they sleep in the most. Often times, people forget though that a bedroom is a room like any other, you have trained yourself to associate it with simply just sleep due to how often you rest there.

Sometimes people will use their bedroom for other things though such as watching television, playing computer games, or even working. While this may seem like a good use for a room on the surface. In all actuality, you're harming yourself by doing this. As I mentioned earlier often times you begin to grow used to the idea of sleeping in that designated spot. This because you sleep their often, go to that room when you get tired, and then promptly fall asleep. Well when you begin to do other activities in your bedroom that are not connected to sleep, what can begin to happen is that you recondition your brain to associate your bedroom not with sleep but wakefulness.

This can lead to you finding it exceedingly difficult to get to sleep at night when you go to your bedroom. While yes, it is convenient to be able to do a wide variety of different tasks all in the same room. It is much less convenient to be unable to sleep when you need it most.

The solution to this problem is quite simple though. Do what you absolutely must in the bedroom and try to relegate other tasks that you know will keep you up, to other rooms. By combining things like avoiding screens before bed. As to not stimulate your brain too much before trying to catch some shut-eye. With useful techniques like calming exercises before preparing for bed.

You can allow yourself to re-establish a healthy sleep cycle which will in turn help diminish the amount of overthinking that you find yourself engaging in during each day. Simply try to remember your sleeping as a habit. You can develop multiple bad habits for your sleep that will all feed into each other and become a compounding problem. Or you can choose to break those habits and to replace them with healthier habits to allow you to get the most sleep you can. While also allowing you to decrease how much time you spend overthinking. Doing all of these things together allows you to avoid one of the major causes of overthinking. And to hopefully break that vicious cycle.

Not getting enough sleep can harm you in a variety of ways. The main way lack of sleep can damage you is in how it negatively affects your mental wellbeing and becomes a compounding problem.

When we do not get a whole lot of sleep our mental health can begin to decline. As a result of our mental health beginning to become more strained, we ourselves can find that we are perhaps performing less well in a wide variety of life areas. This is quite a simple result of being tired.

Think about it if you are tired all the time it is very easy for you to start falling behind on all kinds of different tasks. From not performing well at work. To even the more dangerous such as driving while tired which can sometimes lead to dangerous car accidents. Nowadays people tend to sacrifice their sleep to try and get more work done. With their thinking being that if they can put more work in one day then as a result, they will have less to do the next day. While this kind of idea can seem quite excellent in theory the problem with this thinking arises is the fact that it makes you end up doing actually less work than you normally would. This is because while yes, you are completing a task that if not completed will get delegated to being done the next day. You end up more exhausted in the end when you try to do your goals. If you are tired and exhausted when you are working, then you will not get as much done. In a way, this kind of thinking ends up making you less productive in the end. This can seem like a hard thing to avoid. But you can, in fact, avoid it by fixing your sleep cycle.

One of the often under looked issues with having a poor sleep habit. Is the fact that the worse your sleep is the harder it will become to actually go about getting good sleep? Think back to how sleep is a habit and how the activities you engage in before sleeping and when you are getting read somewhat determine how you will sleep.

Well if you are getting to sleep at a very late hour every night and then getting up even later. What begins to happen is your internal clock starts to get thrown off. You begin to reach a point where that becomes your new normal. This is not a good thing to have happen as this as an issue will only begin to compound itself more and more.

As a result, you can find it difficult to break this habit. Getting to bed at a very late time, for example when the sun begins to rise is the inverse of how we normally sleep. For the most part, our body is used to going to bed when the sun and the associated light generated by it begins to fade out. And is wired to get up when we begin to detect that light again. As a result of throwing that cycle off, you can develop worse sleep.

Now sleep is heavily associated with mental health but why is that? Well, when we get to sleep our brain is developing the resources it needs to get us through the next day, while also storing memories in the places that they need to go. Say for instance you had a stressful day at work and a lot of bad things happened to you. When you start to get ready for sleep and then finally get to sleep this allows your mind some time off from constantly worrying about these kinds of issues. This, in turn, leads to better mental health and those kinds of issues getting placed on the back burner.

Well, when you start to sleep poorly you can't destress properly. As a result, your mind ends up repeating the same scenario over and over again to the point that it is very uncomfortable for you to go through. This can make getting to sleep when you need an even more difficult challenge since if you are stressed out it is more challenging to go to sleep due to you having undue stress that you're going through.

As a result of having this extra stress, it is then more challenging to get to sleep again. This becomes a compounding issue, which only serves to make overthinking and anxiety even worse. As a result of this, your mental health can begin to deteriorate, which is not good.

The final issue that can develop due to a lack of adequate sleep are some of the physical problems that come as a result of it.

When we sleep things like our heart rate, respiration and blood pressure begin to drop, this is done by our body so we begin to feel sleepy, and also give some of our organs a break and allow them to break down toxins.

Well when we do not get the kind of sleep, we need our organs can rest and break down toxins. This can lead to a myriad of issues because dangerous levels of stress hormones can begin to develop. In the short term, these issues are not too damaging but it is the long term that matters.

Things like heart disease can begin to develop as a result. Your heart needs a break and sleep allows it to get this break it needs.

Additionally, if you do not sleep well you tend to become more stressed out as a result. Well, a high level of stress is not good for you and also puts undue stress on your heart. When this happens, you can begin to not feel well physically, we all know of the kind of strange exhaust that comes with being overtired. Well, this kind of crummy feeling is often the result of too many stress hormones being present in our body and as a result us not feeling all too well.

Overthinking can affect more people than just you.

Often times when you overthink you can end up taking out the emotions that this builds up in you out on those you love the most. This is especially true if you work a stressful job where you find yourself being unable to let go after work.

This is pretty common in today's world with people more often than not working multiple jobs to make ends meet. This process of overthinking about work usually stems from a positive place, in the sense that you are trying to complete a task so decide to dedicate a lot of thought and effort into it to try and get it completed.

By doing this to such an extent thought you end up damaging yourself more than you actually make your job easier. Because of you beings stressed you end up not focusing on your job as well as you perhaps could.

So, what ends up inevitably happening is when you go home after a long day of work you find yourself drained and exhausted so the family members and loved ones who you usually enjoy spending time with.

You end up becoming thorns in your side as a result of this.

Your children asking you questions about how your day went ends up becoming a reminder of how stressful your work is and just continues to perpetuate the cycle. As a result of this stress, you can find yourself lashing out at loved ones even when you normally would not mean to.

This lashing out is not done because you dislike your family but because anything else added to your plate ends up feeling like it is going to end up stressing you out more. This is never a healthy thing to have happen to you. And in the end, becomes a further cause of stress.

Because now while also dealing with the stress and tension you are bringing home from your work you are also dealing with the stress of your family being displeased with your current behavior. This is never a good thing, you may find yourself having to have awkward conversations with loved ones over how you have been acting recently. And in the worst cases, this can lead to damage and even the end of certain relationships such as marriages and partners.

So how do you go about ensuring that you leave your stress at the door and do not bring it with you? Well, one thing to remember is that often times we can have trouble changing our mindset day today.

After leaving work it can become quite easy to maintain that same work-related mindset and continue being stressed over what is going on. This is a result of overthinking. See your brain is spending so much time trying to prepare for work and get it finished that you begin to develop tunnel vision. As a result of this tunnel vision, you can start to find it challenging to complete your tasks and get things done the way they need to be completed, especially tasks relating to your familial unit.

To go about de-stressing and removing this tension from work one of the things you can begin to do. Is perhaps allowing yourself some time to de-stress right before you go home. If you have a place that a lot of your coworkers like to frequent after work. Try going to that location and blowing off some steam instead of always letting it follow you home.

Often times you may find yourself in a rush to get back home and do the next thing on your list for the sake of your family. But if you are in a foul mood around your family one of the best things you can do to ensure you do good by them is to go about letting yourself unwind and relax before you begin interacting with them again. This may seem like a challenging thing to do at first, but besides just trying to relax with your coworkers. You can even use this as an opportunity to introduce more beneficial things and habits in your life.

Take going to the gym, for instance, working out has many benefits for both your mind and body. When you exercise your body gets out the energy that has been pent up in it for such a long time. And so, does your mind. You begin to unwind and destress while also reaping many rewards. By trying to find a way to introduce this kind of calm to your life on a regular basis you set yourself up for times where you can just relax and mellow out. Your family will begin to notice the difference as well.

While you can use the time, you have in between commuting as a time to de-stress. Via doing activities you enjoy before heading straight home you can also try and use calming techniques as soon as you get home if this is not an option. This means instead of sitting right down and spending time with your family, try perhaps taking a shower and meditating right after to allow yourself to calm down and mellow out at home.

This is perhaps the best way to go about doing this because you can get back to your loved ones sooner. And also allow yourself to de-stress at your house. When you de-stress at your house what can begin to happen is instead of perhaps associating your home with extra stress you may begin to find that because you practice these calming routines right after your work. You begin to associate the end of work with a calming period. Instead of a time of stress.

Now that you have a newfound understanding of how overthinking functions. Such as how it can cause your mind to become cluttered with all kinds of thoughts you do not need. Leading to you having issues making the proper decisions that you need to, and also how this can cause further issues with overthinking.

You are now better able to combat overthinking in itself. See overthinking has become especially prevalent in today's fast-paced society and as a result of this many people have become afflicted by the many facets of this problem. As you read earlier in the book overthinking is a habitual problem. One that begins as a small little issue but will continue to expand and grow as time goes on. As a result, this problem can become difficult to change and feel like a huge burden that you have to carry.

Conclusion

But you now know-how.

Having read this book besides having learned that overthinking is habitual.

You have begun to now understand that overthinking can come from a wide variety of areas in our life. Most importantly how things like having a boor sleep habits can affect and even make existing overthinking worse.

By understanding this problem at the basic level, you are much more likely to avoid encountering the many different issues that are associated with overthinking. See because overthinking functions as a habit it can seem at first very challenging to break that said habit.

But now you should understand how to break bad habits.

By eliminating things that cause a negative influence on your life you can further yourself. We all know that there are many things in our lives that can have a negative influence on us. But trying to break this influence is often a challenging ordeal, many times we find that in trying to break a bad habit we can sometimes end up developing a worse habit as a result.

This is where understanding the basics of habitual behavior comes from if you do not understand how a habit is formed and how it can play into overthinking you are going to be doomed to continue the process of overthinking. Knowing how a negative influence can cause you to overthink and how as a result your thoughts can begin to become cluttered allows you to take the high road out. When viewing overthinking just as anxiety what can begin to happen is that you will get this black and white view of it.

This misses the many nuances that are associated with it, something as complex as our mind is not going to work in such a simple paradigm it is going to be influenced by many different factors, and this is the case for something like overthinking.

Finally, with learning how meditation works you now have the best defense against overthinking that you can ask for, a time-tested method that has been used by people all around the globe for generations to combat their anxieties and worries. That is what meditation is in the most simple and short definition it is not some kind of esoteric practice, it is a simple calming method. With all of these tools now at your disposal, you are better prepared than ever to combat against overthinking.

Listening To My Body

A practical guide to finding mindfulness, understanding your emotions and developing emotional resilience

By Dr. Belinda Hollis

Introduction

"Mens sana in corpore sano". This is the famous Latin phrase for "a healthy mind in a healthy body" and the main concept of the Hippocrates philosophy. Hippocrates is the father of medicine, so he surely knows what he is talking about. Nowadays, most people do not have the time or the knowledge to listen to what their body is saying. The reality of the matter is that your mind listens to your body and your body listens to your mind. For example, if we feel bad about the way we look or we think we are facing problems with a dietary plan we are following right now are all thoughts and worries that start in our mind. Our body takes on these bad thoughts and the hidden beliefs that are behind those thoughts and you may either suffer from a reduced appetite or an enhanced one.

There are many models and people who suffer from anorexia and when they look at their bodies in the mirror, they get sad or depressed because they think that either their bodies are not beautiful or that they don't deserve this body perfection. Our bodies are composed of cells and each and every one of them "knows" whenever you are sad, happy, angry, displeased, etc.

Our bodies hold and protect our life if something goes wrong with it, then things may not end up well for us. Listening to them is not that hard and it is completely different than you needing your body to be healthy. For example, if you don't ask the help of an expert, you may think that by cutting off all the things that you deem unhealthy and eat only a specific type of food, you will keep your body healthy. This is not the case and this is the reason we must gather every piece of information available on how we can be healthy, if we can't visit an expert, and unnecessarily place our health in danger.

Many people follow strict diets wanting to lose weight. The problem with this way is that when you are so focused on counting calories and how many steps you walked this week, you will be unhappy because you will not listen to your body and your mind which may have given you signs of how wrong this situation was such as hunger pains and unhappiness. Why people gain weight when they are finished with strict diets? Because when the diet is over, they think they are free to do whatever they couldn't do during the time they spend imprisoned in a strict diet.

In this book we will explore how you can successfully listen to your body through many practices such as meditation, mindfulness and many more, and explore the signs of certain serious conditions that could help you avoid letting the symptoms get worse and the problems of following a strict diet on your body and training methods that will keep you healthy.

In the first chapter, we will analyze what are strict diets and the effects they have on a physical and psychological level since they are the number one threat that prevents you from listening to your body due to the fact that they promise a complete makeover. We will also analyze the signs your body sends you on various common conditions such as lactose intolerance to provide you with some useful hints on what it means to listen to your body. In the second chapter, we will examine how meditation will help you in listening to your body. Also, we will analyze everything that is important to understand about meditation that will help beginners in their first steps at the practice as well as present you with numerous basic exercises, to begin with. In the third chapter, we will introduce you to the benefits of mindfulness and how it can help you with your task of listening to your body effectively.

In the fourth chapter, we will provide you with the necessary information about the seven chakras that exist in our bodies and how you could use them to achieve the desired result. In the fifth chapter, we will talk about Somatic Mindfulness and Meditation along with Kundalini Meditation and the tools they are able to provide to reach your goals. In the sixth chapter, we will present you with the necessary information on how to develop your emotional resilience and how to maintain it. Finally yet importantly, in the seventh chapter, we will provide you with the necessary information to develop your self-regulation skills as well as everything you need to know to maintain them. Let us start our journey then! And then, if you like it, I would me more than happy if you could share your thought with a review on Amazon website.

Chapter 1: The Signs Your Body Sends You: Strict Diets and Common Conditions

Dieting has been an integral part of people's quest on how to lose those extra pounds they have gained. Counting how many calories each food you eat has, keeping notes of everything that goes into your mouth, and choosing to follow a strict diet almost always has the exact opposite effect of losing and maintaining the lost weight on a long-term scale. Dieting and eating healthy are opposite.

Many people choose to follow diets, they do so because they actually work but in the short term. They are most appropriate for people who have reached completely unhealthy levels of weight, and those people need to lose a certain percentage of fat in order to avoid any possible fatal danger and when the dieting is over to start eating healthy and maintain a healthy lifestyle.

The good news is that according to studies, fewer and fewer people follow diets and start eating healthy instead, mainly because they have learned their lessons from mistakes of the past. People all over the world have started to understand that if your plan to lose weight does not seem possible to maintain for long, then you shouldn't even bother starting in the first place.

But how would you know if your diet is bad for you? By learning to listen to your body and the signs it sends you whenever your diet is wrong and it needs to be changed immediately. Those signs vary from subtle to downright obvious, but they will always be there since the plan of your diet will influence your body on a much bigger scale than you could ever imagine. What we place inside our bodies will affect your skin, your mind, and how productive you are during the day.

There are not a few cases of people whose diet and their body shows them that their diet is not appropriate for their health. Let us see all those signs that your body tells you to stop this dietary plan and start eating healthy.

One sign of bad dietary plans is bad breath caused by Ketosis, the result of metabolic process that happens when glucose, a source of energy, is not enough in our bodies and our metabolism burns fat. This results in creating acids named "ketones" that can make your breath smell bad. People who follow low carb diets are more prone to accumulate ketones to their breath and these diets and ketones can be extremely dangerous for people that have type 1 diabetes. They should visit a doctor due to the fact that ketones may mean that there is not enough insulin in their bodies. The problem will be resolved if you increase your eating portions so that the required energy you need is taken through food. On the other hand, bad breath can be caused also from smoking, coffee, and by not caring for your teeth enough.

If your hair is thinning it means that your iron levels are low. Iron is essential to the production of red blood cells and they in turn transfer oxygen throughout our blood. If your iron levels are low, you may feel sluggish and your hair will get thinner. Eating green vegetables such as broccoli and spinach, and red meat will enhance your iron levels. For women, iron levels could fall even further due to menstruation and not only due to bad diet programs, so they should follow a dietary plan which is full in iron.

If you notice that you suffer from continual diarrhea, you may have Coeliac disease. Coeliac disease is a reaction of our immune system from eating gluten found in barley, wheat, and rye. Our small intestine is triggered by eating gluten and can lead to weight loss, abdominal pain, and diarrhea. If you cut off gluten from your dietary plan, the problem will be resolved and keep in mind that Coeliac disease is completely different from gluten intolerance even though they have the same symptoms.

If you feel constipated, it is your body's way of telling you that you are not drinking enough water and your diet is lacking in fiber. For regular and normal bowel movement, both water and fiber are needed since the fiber is able to attract water which in turn transfers it in the body in an easier way. In such cases, drink more water and at the same time add to your diet high fiber foods, like whole grains, nuts, beans, and dried fruit.

If you feel constantly tired and that your energy levels are low, there is a high chance that you are taking into your body too much sugar. Too much sugar or other carbohydrates can make you feel tired all the time and for you to have low energy levels. This happens because the sugar will raise the insulin that is in your body at first, but if you have a daily intake of more sugar than necessary; it will cause your energy levels to fall. Don't make the mistake of believing that when you feel less energetic it is right to eat more sugar. On the contrary, reduce your sugar and your energy will elevate and stabilize in no time.

If you are going to the toilet frequently to release fluid, you are dehydrated. Often people think the opposite is true, but even if when you drink too much water, your bladder is full and triggers the brain signaling you that it is time to relieve yourself, this is not always the case. Your bladder may also be irritated by your urine is concentrated in one specific location. The solution to this problem is to drink much more water in order for your urine to be clearer than yellow.

If you constantly feel as if you are swollen all the time, this is a sure sign of your following a bad diet plan. If you feel gassy, especially after eating dairy products, you might even be lactose intolerant. There are signs that will tell you if you suffer from this condition such as nausea, vomiting, gas, diarrhea and cramps in the abdomen area that will begin from thirty minutes to two hours after eating anything that contains lactose. Lactose intolerance is happening due to the fact that lactase, an enzyme that is produced in our small intestine, is insufficient in our bodies.

Even though many people exist, whose lactase levels are low and have no problems in digesting dairy products without any problems, there are also those who face the mentioned symptoms after they eat dairy foods. In this case, the lactose contained in the food you eat is directly transferred into the colon without first being processed and absorbed. When it reaches the colon, undigested lactose is coming in contact with normal bacteria, resulting in the signs of lactose intolerance.

When you are always hungry at the end of the day by following a specific diet, then you are not following the right diet for you and your body suffers along with you. After a day of successfully following your diet plan, night time is another matter. You may be so hungry that even your willpower is not strong enough to keep you from a bag of chips. Eating excessively is caused by your body's demand that it doesn't get all the necessary nutrients needed to be full and healthy. Keep in mind that a proper diet with the purpose of being healthy and right for people, should not eliminate food groups unless it is necessary for medical reasons.

A psychological sign of you following the wrong diet plan is if you are constantly in a bad mood. Food cravings will irritate you when you are trying to cut down your carbs and calories. Also, the sugar in your blood is low during this process, a fact that contributes to severe mood swings.

Research has shown that diets consisting of low carb consumption can have a severe effect on your thyroid, which is responsible for the temperature of your body. If your thyroid slows down, you will feel cold even during summer. Try not to cut down all carbs. Just make certain that you include in your diet complex carbs such as whole grain bread, and more other foods like pasta.

Another sure sign of an unhealthy diet is wrinkles and acne. Diets that are lacking vitamin A will have a huge impact on your skin since vitamin A has an essential role in controlling the production of retinoid. Any deficiency caused to this nutrient could also drive you to have brittle nails and dry hair. To solve this problem, eat foods that are rich in vitamin A such as carrots or sweet potatoes.

Mental illnesses may stem from a bad and unbalanced diet. If you feel depressed all the time, you may follow a diet that is not providing you enough minerals, vitamins and Omega-3 acids. Your mood can be changed by taking nutritional supplements with vitamin B12. They are usually prescribed to patients that are trying to tackle mental illnesses.

Memory can also be affected by eating badly. According to researches, saturated fats had an effect on women who showed lower memory abilities and were slower on thinking tests when compared to those women that did not eat those saturated fats. If you want a sharp memory, you should do well to avoid fast food and French fries.

Our immune system is also affected by a bad diet. For example, you may always be sick if you follow a low-protein diet since proteins help you by reinforcing your immune system. If you ban essential nutrients of your body, you will weaken your immune system and therefore you will leave yourself open to illnesses. Make sure to stay healthy and eat many proteins such as lean meats, and beans.

When you have a small cut or even a larger injury, you may have noticed that it takes more time to heal than the time it takes on other people. For a wound to heal fast and appropriately, it requires a considerable amount of nutrients to be in your body, so if you heal slowly it may be due to the fact that your nutrients are not enough to help through the process. A bad diet can and will affect the resilience of the new tissue, the time you will need to recover from a wound, no matter how small it is, as well as how effectively your body will battle an infection that may affect the wound. Research has shown that proper amounts of protein, nutrients, and calories are needed for wounds to be healed effectively.

The above are signs of the physical kind your body is showing you to indicate that something is really wrong with your diet and your overall health. However, our body includes our mind and hence the emotional responses to a bad lifestyle. We mentioned how depression can be enhanced by strict diets and generally following a bad lifestyle. This can also happen when it comes to anxiety. Although your way of eating is not scientifically proven that can cause an anxiety disorder, it may make the symptoms of anxiety worse. Strict diets for weight loss may lead you to anxious moods as well as restricting calories along with proteins. Also, overeating will cause the same effects because it will lead to weight gain. Eating too little or too much will increase your anxiety due to the fact that you will never be satisfied with the ending result. A balanced diet will resolve this problem since you will see the desired results in your body as well as in your emotional responses.

Anxiety disorder can be revealed through physical symptoms that will warn you of the condition. There are many types of anxiety disorders such as panic disorders, separation anxiety, generalized anxiety disorder, phobias, social anxiety, and obsessive-compulsive disorder that have unique symptoms linked to fears that each type of anxiety can produce. Generally, anxiety disorders have many common physical symptoms and your body will express them to warn you of the danger.

These signs include nausea, stomach pains, digestive trouble, tiredness and fatigue, sleep issues such as insomnia, headaches, shortness of breath or rapid breathing, sweating, increased heart rate, muscle pain or tension, shaking or trembling. For example, if you are going through a panic attack you may feel dizzy, develop chest pain, have trouble breathing, and feel as if you are choking, or feel as though you may pass out.

Keep in mind that anxiety is how the body responds to stress and alerts you to potential threats that you should be prepared to deal with. For example, you may breathe faster due to the fact that your lungs are trying to take in more oxygen just in case the need arises to escape from a situation.

Stress can also be caused by bad eating habits. People who follow a strict diet are more prone to develop emotional stress than those who follow a balanced diet. Fewer calories and carbohydrates are likely to multiply stress since both are essential for the brain to work correctly as well as to produce a number of chemicals that make people feel good, like serotonin. However, eating more food than is necessary for our bodies can also enhance stress because we gain weight and therefore we may get depressed by our image and stress out to lose this extra weight by following strict and unbalanced diets.

What happens when we suffer from depression? What are the physical symptoms that warn us of this disorder? Most people are aware of the emotional symptoms, but our bodies react to depression too so as to warn us of the dangers we are placing ourselves into. Depression causes constant and persistent emotions of sadness and a lack of interest in things about your life that you previously loved. This is the main reason why depression is a dangerous mood disorder since it can lead you to think that life is not worth living anymore.

The physical symptoms of depression include back pain and headaches that if they existed before as migraines they will probably get worse. Also, you will endure chest pain, but it may also occur due to a serious lung, heart, stomach condition. You may also have diarrhea or be constipated for long periods of time. Added to this, you will feel tired as if getting out of bed is an impossible task, no matter how much sleep you get.

However, people who suffer from depression, are not able to sleep as well as they did before. They may not even be able to fall asleep once they retire for the night or wake up too early while other people may sleep much more than they normally did, before developing depression. Last but not least, depressed people will notice a change in their appetite which will result in either losing weight or gain weight. The result is different for every person.

The above are some of the signs our bodies will show us when we follow a bad diet, when we have lactose intolerance, when we have anxiety or when we suffer from depression. What happens though, when our body has to warn us that our overall health? How will your body tell you that you need to make different lifestyle choices and take care of it more? There are signs that will show you when the time has come to take responsibility for your body and start listening to it.

Your skin will show you if you take care of your health appropriately. With the exception of people who are diagnosed with skin issues such as acne, bad skin will tell the tale of your overall state of health. If you keep seeing blemishes or stretch marks, it can be the result of a bad diet or lack of a daily skincare routine and cleanliness.

Sleep is extremely important for following a healthy lifestyle and if you are not able to sleep at night, there can be many reasons for this occurrence such as getting less caffeine, following a bad dietary plan, and not letting out much energy during the day that prevents you from falling asleep. Eight hours of sleep a day is required for us to stay healthy and productive throughout our lives. Pinpoint the problems that are causing your body to refuse to get the rest it needs and make the necessary changes.

Low vitamin levels can be expressed through constantly chapped lips, bad fingernails and toenails or skin problems. If you have to always apply lip balm in order for your lips to seem healthy, then you need a vitamin boost. Make the necessary changes to your diet and when you get the appropriate nutrients, you will notice your lips improving too.

Usually, chapped lips indicate a deficiency of vitamin B-2 or else riboflavin. This vitamin is necessary for healthy nails, skin, and hair. You can get vitamin B-2 by eating dairy products, vegetables, eggs, nuts, beans, and lean meats. Adult males need 1.3 milligrams of vitamin B-2 while adult females need 1.0 milligrams of vitamin B-2 in their system.

Another vitamin your body needs and when not found in appropriate numbers in your system may cause chapped lips, skin problems or swollen tongue is vitamin B-3 or else niacin. To receive the needed amount of 13 to 20 milligrams of vitamin B-3 per day, you need to eat foods such as beef, poultry, tune, been, milk, vegetables, and halibut. An insufficient amount of vitamin B-6 or else pyridoxine can also be a sign of skin problems and cracks found at the corners of your mouth. Adult women and men up to 50 years of age should receive 1.3 milligrams of vitamin B-6 every day from food such as legumes, meats, green vegetables, and whole grains.

Another physical sign your body shows that you are not healthy is cold feet and hands. Even though the environment you live in may be the cause, if you constantly feel that your hands and feet are cold, it may be considered as a sign of cardiovascular problems, specifically circulation issues. In other words, there is not enough blood flowing in certain places in your body.

Another sign you should watch out for is if you have noticed that you are getting shorter. As we age, it is normal to lose our height, but when this is happening earlier than is considered normal and in extremely small amounts, it can be a sign of a serious health problem such as bone loss. Another condition that can be attributed to this situation is not receiving enough essential nutrients such as calcium and protein. In the long term, this condition may lead to loss of the density of the bones and fractures.

When your legs swell, it may be a way of your body saying that there may be a problem with your kidney, heart or thyroid condition. Thyroid problems are also indicated through your neck swelling and specifically, your thyroid may be overactive when your neck swelling happens out of the blue and at an extreme speed.

For women, dark and coarse hairs that grow on the chin may be a sign of polycystic ovary syndrome. There is a hormonal anomaly that can also affect a woman's period and thus a woman's fertility. Other signs of polycystic ovary syndrome are skin issues from enhanced levels of androgens, irregular period, and weight gain at the area around the stomach, trouble sleeping, depression and/or anxiety, and ovarian cysts.

Also, if your big toe looks swollen and you haven't injured it in any way, it could be a sign and an early symptom of gout. Gout is extremely painful and can place you at the risk of developing chronic diseases such as kidney disease and elevated blood pressure. Another sign of gout is swollen joints, so if you notice these two symptoms happening for prolonged periods of time, a visit to your doctor is necessary.

When you wake up and you still feel exhausted, it may be a physical sign of restless leg syndrome, in other words, we wake up still feeling tired because our bodies never truly entered a relaxed state during the night. You may also have noticed an urge of moving your legs, especially when you sit down. A visit to your doctor will surely be a good move since he or she will point you in the right direction.

If you notice that you are sweating through your clothes and specifically on your underarms, face, or hands, you may have hyperhidrosis. It can be a sign of a medical condition, for example, an overactive thyroid, even though the sweat is harmless. If you also experience weight loss, fever, or shortness in your breath, you should visit your doctor due to the fact that there are several medical reasons for your excess sweating such as lung or heart disease. You should start immediately by changing your diet and cut back on spicy food, curries, and garlic.

Also, if you notice skin tags appearing in high numbers, it could be a sign of type 2 diabetes. They are caused by insulin-like growth factor 1 that is a protein commonly found in diabetes and can arouse skin overgrowth. If you also notice yellow bumps on your glutes, feet, joints, and hands it may be a warning of fat concentration under your skin. These spots are called xanthomas and are a warning that your blood fats such as cholesterol are extremely high. Another condition they can indicate is diabetes, some types of cancers, and pancreatitis.

Last but not least, snoring is a common sign of sleep apnea that is linked with an increased risk of heart disease. Snoring is also linked to thickening carotid arteries in the neck and such damage can lead to heart attack and stroke. Studies have shown that snoring is found more commonly to people that smoke, have high cholesterol or are overweight.

If you push yourself and overdo it with your body, you might end up exhausted and do more harm to your body than good. If you don't listen to what your body has to say, how will you know what it needs and what should you do in order for you to live a healthy and long life?

Don't be fooled by today's world. You may be busy and postpone your visit to the doctor since you think any symptom your body shows, will pass. You don't care about following a healthy and balanced diet because straining your body will get you the desired results faster, so how you look is the only thing that matters.

Keep in mind that your body will help you and be there for you if you take care of it. Your body is the house of your soul and it needs to be cared for as you take care of the house you live in. If your body thrives, you will thrive. If your body is healthy, you will be healthy. When we visit the doctor, we do so because we saw something. We noticed something was not going well within our body. So, how could you start forging this bond with your body? How can you start listening to it?

Chapter 2: How to Listen to Your Body: Meditation

In the previous chapter, we mentioned the different conditions and problems your body is trying to warn you about, but many people do not know how to listen to the cues and others choose to ignore them because circumstances may suite this choice. However, it is imperative to master the necessary skills that will help you listen to your body and prevent further dangers to your health and general well-being.

The prevalent way of you being able to listen to everything your body needs to tell you is through meditation. But what is meditation? Meditation an exercise for the mind that includes ways to focus, relax, and be aware of everything around you. Think of this as the equivalent of physical exercise but for the mind, not the body. The definition of meditation according to psychology is "a family of mental training practices that are designed to familiarize the practitioner with specific types of mental processes".

Meditation is often done by a single person, in a seated position with the eyes closed even if it is practiced from a group of people, usually in cases of a meditation retreat. Also, meditation is practiced through keeping your body completely still and your eyes closed even though there are practices such as Zazen and Trataka that let you keep your eyes open. This practice is extremely effective and helps you with your observation. In open monitoring meditation, you will be focusing on the environment around you in the present, allowing no disturbances or focusing only on one thing. In focused meditation that helps you with concentration, you will be focused on only one object. Meditation also helps you with your awareness levels that keep you focused on the present moment and you will pay attention to neither focusing nor observing anything.

Initially, meditation derived from the word "meditate" which means thinking strongly about something. All that changed as time passed until meditation came to mean what it does today, focusing your attention on thinking deeply. For instance, according to Christianity, meditation is a form of a reflective prayer that helps people create a bond with God or lets them think in peace, their religious beliefs. According to Buddhism, meditation is one out of the three methods that purify the mind and can lead to the achievement of Nirvana.

So, in this case, with meditation, the goal for you is to achieve focusing and listening to your body. There are many meditation techniques to choose from and to find the one that corresponds better to your needs, you should try them all, practice each one for a week, and in the end conclude which one attains the best results for your goal. According to scientists, there are two categories of meditation that are based on how you focus your attention.

In Focused Attention meditation, you will turn your attention on only one object for the duration of the practice. The object you will focus on is not necessarily a physical object. It can also be your breath, part of your body, images in your mind or a mantra. As you practice more and gain experience, you will be able to focus longer on the object of your choice and external distractions will be less frequent and shorter in time. In Open Monitoring meditation, your focus is not turned into only one object, but you will keep it spread on all parts of your experience, with no attachments. You will be able to acknowledge all your thoughts, memories, feelings and all sounds or scents from your environment.

Zen or Zazen meditation comes from Chinese Zen Buddhism and its origins can be traced to the 6th century CE. Zazen means "seated meditation" in Japanese since you will find it practiced more commonly seated on the floor with your legs crossed. To all types of meditation, posture is extremely important. You can meditate when seated on the floor on a cushion or on a chair. Your spine should be totally straight all through your lower back, up towards your neck and you should not lean on anything. This is also the case for Zazen meditation. You will have to keep your mouth closed and your eyes barely open, resting your gaze at the ground that is close to you.

Zazen positions vary and the simplest one is Burmese Position, in which your legs are crossed and your feet are resting on the floor. The Half Lotus position is the one where your left foot is found onto the right thigh and the right leg is hidden under. In Full Lotus position, each foot is put on the opposite thigh. There is also the Seiza Position where you kneel on the floor with your buttocks resting on the heels of your feet.

During Zazen meditation, you can turn your whole attention to your breath, going inside you through the nose. Inhale and start counting from 10 backward for all the duration of the inhale and exhale process. When you reach number 1, start over again from 10 and in case you become distracted and get confused while counting, bring your attention back to ten and start over again. In Zazen meditation, breath is vital, the most important activity of the human body. Breath is one with the mind because when your mind is restless your breath is affected too by being agitated.

Another thing you can do during Zazen meditation is Shikantaza or else just sitting. In this form, you will not fix your focus on only one thing such as your breath, but you will try to stay in the present moment by being aware and noticing all the thoughts that pass through your mind while at the same time you do not ponder on anything.

Mantra meditation revolves around the mantra that is a word or a sentence without necessarily any particular meaning that the one who practices meditation repeats for focusing his or her mind. A mantra is not something used as a way for you to convince yourself that something needs to be done or is true. Teachers of meditation argue about the usage of mantra. Some say that the words used in a mantra as well as the correct spelling are extremely important because the sound of the phrase or word and the meaning have a vibration and the practitioner should be eased into a mantra. Some others say that a mantra is only the tool used for the said person to focus his or her mind and the choice of words is not relevant to the purpose of meditation.

You can also find Mantra meditation called "Om meditation" since that is the usual mantra used during the practice. Mantras can be found in Buddhist, Hindu, Tibetan, Taoism, Sikhism, and Jainism traditions. Other mantras that can be used when you practice is "om Namah Shivaya", "so-ham", "om mani Padme hum", "yam", "ham", and "Rama".

In this type of meditation, you are still in a sitting position with your back straight and your eyes are kept closed. You will repeat the mantra of your choice in your mind, without actually speaking the words,

111

continuously until the end of the session. For as long as you keep repeating the mantra, it conjures a vibration in your mind that allows it to become more aware and delve into deeper levels of your awareness. Also, as you keep repeating the mantra, there will be a time when the words will seem indistinct since you will be led into the field of consciousness.

The mantra will aid you to disconnect from your thoughts that keep entering your mind and you will reach a stage where no thought will interrupt your meditation time or the thoughts will be fleeting and as soon as they enter your head, they will leave. If you are not able to achieve this from the start, don't give up. It takes time for people to reach a level such as the above.

You may want to start for the first time by repeating your mantra out loud, to help you get used to it in a better and easier way. As soon as you are comfortable with your mantra, then start whispering it. It can be barely heard and the sound is barely there. Then, you can start saying the mantra inside your head. If you start using your tongue and throat at first, don't think of it as a wrong move. With practice, you will be able to stop moving those muscles and you will reach a level when the mantra will enter your mind without you trying to repeat it.

By repeating the mantra at a fast pace, you will feel energized while when repeating it at a slower pace, your mind will feel and be calm. If you find random thoughts entering your mind that prevent you from reaching your goal, you may want to tune up the mantra. Speak it louder in your head or else your focus will not remain and instead you will be overwhelmed by troubled thoughts. Added to this, you can repeat the mantra whenever you inhale and exhale. You could also repeat it two times when inhaling and when exhaling. It all depends on how you feel and with what option you are more comfortable, for example, you could repeat the mantra by giving no thought to breathing.

According to research, people find it easier to maintain their focus while using a mantra than when they try to focus solely on their breathing. This is happening because when you repeat words into your mind, thoughts, sound, memories, and sensations are not that easy to interrupt you. You will be focused on your mantra, something that provides you with relaxation and awareness. You can also choose a mantra that means something to you. You want to start listening to your body, so you should use a word that makes you comfortable enough to attain this goal.

Walking meditation is another way for you could become more aware of your body. It is not as simple as taking a walk on the street since it is done at a much slower pace than usual walks and it requires focusing on our breath or other objects. In walking meditation your eyes are open, your body is in a standing position and it moves, and you will be more in contact with the world outside. Since your body will be moving, you will be more aware of the sensations that flow through your body and also, you will be more grounded to the present.

When trying to choose a place for walking meditation, you need to keep in mind that you should practice it somewhere that is far from traffic and extremely populated areas. The place where you will be walking should not make you too distracted by the scenery so that your mind is able to be focused to meditate. At first, walking meditation may seem a bit strange, so it would be better if you practiced at your backyard or somewhere else that makes you feel comfortable.

The perfect length for walking meditation is at least fifteen minutes. It is easier to practice for more than a few minutes since you will not be seated or required to stay still. The slower you walk the better it will be for your focus. If you can't focus or you feel tense, try to walk even slower up until you are able to focus and ground yourself to the present moment. Before you start walking, it would be better if you try to connect with your body first by standing up and still while taking deep breaths.

Have your feet hip-width apart and let your weight fall evenly on both legs. The moment you feel stabilized on the ground, take a few deep breaths and let your eyes close. Then, focus on your body and try to feel everything, for example, how your body feels while you stand still and become aware of all the sensations that are flowing inside you. Even how the air feels on your hands is considered as being aware of your body. As far as walking meditation is concerned we have several techniques to choose from.

The Theravada Walking Meditation is an integral part of Buddhist tradition when training. Many monks that reside in monasteries in Thailand walk for hours each day, developing their concentration. If you want to practice Theravada Walking Meditation, you have to pick a straight path with a distance of approximately thirty to forty feet. If you are able to walk it barefoot, it is highly recommended, but you can also wear light, comfortable shoes. Your back should be straight and your eyes lowered so as to when you walk, your attention should be focused on your feet.

Feel your legs muscles tense as you lift them and then lower them while walking and the sensations you feel through the air touching your whole body. Especially if you are barefoot, feel the sensations of each passing step as your feet come into contact with the ground. You should be aware of every part of your body since each step you take creates new sensations and leaves the old ones behind. When you reach the end of your path, stop, turn around, stop again and start heading back. Walk the path back and forth for as long as you wish and each time note your sensations. If you feel your mind wandering, focus back by asking yourself where you are focused on. During walking meditation, if you feel the need to stop for a moment, then do so, especially if intruding thoughts are too strong for you to not think about. There is no right way of what you should fee. Each person experiences different sensations and emotions when practicing walking meditation. Your goal should be for you to connect with your body and the way it feels when you walk by focusing on each sensation.

Another type of walking meditation is Zen Walking Meditation or Kinhin. In Zen Walking Meditation you will have to walk a path of approximately forty feet long while maintaining a particular posture. It can also be done between breaks of seated meditation. You should stand with your back straight but not tense and your weight should be evenly distributed to each leg. Sense your feet touching the ground and take the Shashu position that is making a fist with your left hand and grasp this fist with your other hand. Start walking the path while maintaining your focus on the movements of your legs and be aware of your mind instructing your body to move.

Your eyes should be lowered so as to not focus on anything and use your sensations to smell the air, hear the sounds of the path you are walking on and when you reach the end of the road, repeat the practice. Your pace should be relevant to the connection of your mind has with your body. For example, if you are tense, your mind may instruct your body to walk at a fast pace, don't try to change it. If your mind is at peace, it will instruct your body to move at a slower pace, don't try to change that either. It would be best to not think of the pace you are walking on while you practice Zen Walking Meditation, let your mind and your body to work that out alone.

There is also Mindfulness Walking Meditation, but this type of walking meditation will be analyzed in later chapters when we will talk about mindfulness as a way to listen to your body. Walking meditation offers a great opportunity for those who want to be more aware of the signs their body is sending them. It helps connect you to your body and mind and also offers you the necessary physical exercise for your body.

Meditation can be practiced whenever you want within the day. However, it is highly recommended to meditate early in the morning as soon as you wake up because the chances of skipping meditation practice later are high and because you will start your day with an open mind. It is also recommended, the place where you will practice meditation to be somewhere that makes you feel comfortable and where there will be as few interruptions as possible. When you practice meditation, your body should not be depleted of energy, so you should better not meditate after exercising your body or after staying for long hours at work. This also means that you shouldn't mediate when you feel the need to sleep and not when you have just eaten; you should wait about two or three hours after eating to mediate.

Before you start your practice session, you have to calm your body and relax it. Try to fill your mind with positive thoughts and emotions and if you find it difficult, remember your goal and try to do the previous two steps again. If during meditation, you get distracted, don't give up, it happens often when you have just started and it is important to feel happy when concentrated because you are letting all negativity go away and you are connecting with both your mind and body. When you are finished meditating, try not to end the session abruptly, instead, try to slowly move your arms, open your eyes, and move your legs.

In order for you to see results from this practice, meditation has to be repeated every day or else the benefits may be short and will not have the depth you'd wish to achieve. You need to search and discover if listening to your body is what you truly wish to achieve in order for you to commit to meditation. If that is your true goal, link it to meditation and think about how it will help you with getting better at listening to your body. Generally, meditation will help you focus, be more observant, and will teach you how to come in touch with all parts of your body.

To further enhance your motivation for practicing meditation, if listening to your body is not enough, there are many health benefits of practicing meditation daily. One of them is that meditation reduces stress and perhaps this is the most common and known reason people decide to start practicing it. When we are mentally and physically stressed this causes elevated production of cortisol, the stress hormone. In turn, this elevated production of cortisol causes the release of chemicals in our body, named cytokines. As a result, we can face problems sleeping, raise the chances of getting anxiety and depression, and contribute to fatigue.

Research has shown that meditation also helps to control anxiety. Since this practice helps us reduce stress, it also helps to better handle anxiety disorders, for example, social anxiety, phobias, and panic attacks. People who work in professions that require a lot of pressure, choose meditation since it can also help reduce the anxiety that has to do with your work environment.

Your emotional health will too be improved since meditation can reduce cytokines that can affect your mood and/or lead to depression. To people who already suffer from depression, fewer cytokines will help them tackle this problem along with the help of their family, friends, and professional help. Meditation also helps you to identify the thoughts that are causing you harm since they may be filled with self-loathing and negativity. It makes you more aware of your thoughts, especially the negative ones, and enables you to leave them behind and turn them into positive ones by fixing the aspects of your life you hated before.

Your attention is increased and you are focused on something for a longer amount of time since you are required in meditation to focus on something whether it is your breathing or a mantra. Added to this, with continued practice of meditation, you develop a mental discipline that may help you fight various addictions you may have. You will enhance your willpower, learn how to control your impulses, and turn your attention to something that is more productive and healthy. You will learn more about yourself and why you intentionally harm yourself by indulging in these addictive behaviors.

If you had any problems sleeping, you will find out that by practicing meditation, your body will relax and therefore let all the tension of the day go, automatically bringing you in a peaceful and calm state which helps you fall asleep and not even wake up during the night by negative thoughts and unresolved problems. The health benefits are numerous and do not only concern listening to your body. Meditation also teaches you how to take care of your body which is essentially an integral part of reading the sign and listening to everything our bodies need to tell us.

Make no mistake believing everything is going to be easy at the beginning. You may feel the urge to give up because you believe that you are doing everything wrong or you don't have time for meditation. Like everything else, meditation needs dedication. Set a time and place during the day and commit to it where you will focus only on practicing meditation. You could even reward yourself each time you complete a meditation session. Keep telling yourself that you are doing this to be healthier and form a bond with your body, something that you didn't have before.

Many people make the mistake of expecting to see immediate results too soon even though they may not practice meditation daily. It should be clear to everyone that decides to start practicing meditation that it should be practiced on a daily basis for you to witness the desired results. To make this point clearer, the length of your practice doesn't matter as much as consistency does. Five or ten minutes of practice every day is way better than an hour for two times each week. This is why most people who practice or teach meditation advise you to start in the morning before starting your daily routine. Even if your schedule is full, you could wake up earlier and practice meditation for three minutes at first if you can't make the session last more.

Many people have the same problem when practicing meditation that have with weight loss. They expect immediate results from the first day. However, you will never experience immediate results on both matters and if you expect to witness any benefits too soon, you will end up giving up in the end. Practice meditation without expecting anything in return, just go for the relaxation it brings and sees it as necessary as taking a shower every day. If you do it just because you expect to be less stressed by the first minute and don't learn how to enjoy it, then there is no point in starting practicing meditation in the first place.

Many meditation sessions fail because you don't prepare yourself before you start. Take a seat or before you start walking wait for a couple of minutes to calm your body and breath, and to connect with your mind. It is just like physical exercise, it is a mistake to start physically working on your body without stretching first. Also, keep in mind that there is a right meditation technique for you since different people are feeling better with different practices. For the first few months, you can evaluate different techniques, for example, you may prefer walking meditation instead of seated meditation, until you find which one is perfect for your personality and goals. If you keep trying different practices for a long amount of time, you may get disappointed because some may have different effects than the ones you actually need. Besides, it is better to find one practice and focus on perfecting it than struggling with learning them all.

Since you care to start meditation, don't make the mistake of thinking if you are doing it right or wrong. You will overanalyze your session during the time when you should be focusing on relaxing and connecting with your mind and body. If you find yourself wondering about this, you will interrupt your session by keeping your mind busy on different things than your actual session. Also, this train of thought will sometimes drain you of the motivation needed to continue the meditation session because you will keep thinking how wrong you are doing it or how unsure you are if you are doing right or not. Just focus on the session and in time you will master the right way of meditating. The only thing two things you need to start is concentration and being aware of when your mind wanders off to irrelevant thoughts.

Another thing you should know for starting meditating is to start learning how to observe your state of mind. If you are plagued with problems that are not serious, such as breaking a cup, meditation will take more than normal to help you. In other words, for meditation to help you, you need to help yourself and not expect for miracles to happen. We are taught how to meditate to keep our minds focused and calm, but if after you finish practicing, you let every little problematic detail into your mind to torture you, almost everything you have accomplished the previous minutes goes in vain. Think of meditation this way. You have been working out in the gym for an hour or two and the rest of the day you are eating junk food and having sugar-filled drinks. Would this help you have a healthier body? No. So, the same principle applies to meditation too.

Meditation will help with your job too. Your mind will be trained in being aware of your task at hand right at the moment that is given to you. You will learn through meditation what are your strengths, weaknesses, and talents. Your stress levels will be reduced and that leaves you with an opportunity to actually enjoy what you are doing without overthinking about certain things related to work. Not to mention that your productivity and work quality will improve since you will be able to schedule and prioritize your responsibilities better since meditation will enhance your self-control.

Also, you could practice meditation with your family. Meditation will have a profound impact on your children's lives since it helps the brain function properly. It can also boost their energy and help kids learn how to keep their attention focused on any task they will be given. Meditation can also help them build kindness and love for themselves and for others. Children are able to learn anything at a faster pace than adults and have higher chances of maintaining the practice of meditation throughout their lives.

There are more types of meditation that will help you develop a deep connection with your body to be able to read the signs that are sent to you. However, they are too important and for this reason, will be analyzed in length in later chapters. For example, mindfulness is another essential part of learning how to listen to your body and is often confused as being the same thing as meditation. They may share some important values, but they also share important differences.

Chapter 3: How to Listen to Your Body: Mindfulness

Many people nowadays have heard of the word mindfulness and how important it is to be mindful. Many also have read that mindfulness and meditation is the same thing. Truth be told, mindfulness is not a new trend and has been present for thousands of years. It can be traced in Eastern religions like Buddhism and Hinduism and modern practitioners of mindfulness in the West have learned it from both the Buddhist and the Hindu tradition.

But what is mindfulness? The definition of mindfulness is the skill to be fully present and aware of the present moment. It is part of meditation that involves focusing your mind on being aware of where you are, what you see, and what you sense right now. There are four foundations of mindfulness that include Body Mindfulness, Sensation Mindfulness, Mind Mindfulness, and Mental Phenomena Mindfulness. As we said earlier, mindfulness and awareness are inherently linked together. But to be aware, you need to meditate since meditation is about awareness too.

The distinction between mindfulness and meditation may be tricky, but one difference is that mindfulness can be practiced everywhere, at any time, and along with anyone, the only thing you have to do in the most simple form of mindfulness is to be focused only on the present moment you enjoy with someone at any place. Also, mindfulness can be practiced during meditation where meditation is only practiced at a certain time schedule and the person practicing it does so individually and in a relatively quiet and calm place.

Mindfulness offers you a better understanding, better health, and emotional recovery while meditation is able to offer all of these and add self-discovery, spiritual and personal growth. All in all, meditation is a pretty big term that encompasses mindfulness since its goal is to achieve the maximum level of concentration and consciousness. So, mindfulness is considered a part of meditation such as yoga, tantra, breathing, and silence.

The benefits of mindfulness will obviously include almost the same benefits meditation has to offer such as low levels of stress by the improvement of emotion regulation, it increases your focus, it helps you when dealing with sleep problems such as insomnia, it aides you in being productive to the workplace, it helps you control your anxiety, it will help you get over your addiction, it helps you relax, it nurtures your ability to feel compassion and it can also help you regulate your blood pressure. So, what do you need to know to practice mindfulness? To start with there are seven Attitudes of Mindfulness that you need to adopt, practice, and follow if you want to achieve true mindfulness.

The first attitude includes you to stop judging others. It is a fact that we live in a world where everything has to be black and white and passing judgments, however small, is taught to us since we were kids. To tackle this problem, start to notice whenever you are passing judgment both on yourself and on others. Try to lessen the times of this happening and you will see as a result that, surprisingly, you will start handling stress better. Passing judgment has its own form of stress; even subconsciously we may feel obligated to judge what someone says or does. Added to this, when we pass judgment on a person, we may wonder if we were right or wrong and if we should feel guilty if we wronged that person. Stressful isn't it?

Another skill/attitude you need to develop is patience which is extremely important for the rest of our life. Through mindfulness, you will realize that you have to let things unfold at their own pace and at their own time. There is no need to rush things or feel anxious whenever something didn't work out. When you are patient, you will no longer linger in the past or wait for the future to come as a child waits for Santa Clause. This happens because people think that their time should be full of activities for their lives to have meaning. Didn't you find yourself in a situation when you needed something so much you spent almost all your money on? Patience teaches us that this is wrong and we should be aware that the right to do something is or isn't that one.

The attitude of the beginner's mind involves our experiences at the present moment. It urges you to perceive everything as you are seeing them for the first time. This allows you to be open to new experiences and opportunities, to be happy for each passing moment you are and to be rest assured that you don't need to know every answer for every problem or question. Due to this mindset, you will become less attached to your past expectations that you have set for people or experiences and you will learn to be aware of many unique possibilities that come your way.

Trust in your feelings as well as in yourself, is the fourth attitude of mindfulness and an essential part of this practice. This part is where you are urged to search inside yourself, to find your insecurities along with your strengths and to tackle your supposed flaws as well as enhance your abilities. You will learn how to take responsibility for yourself and for your life by trusting yourself to make the right choices and if they are not, then you will learn to face your mistakes.

Non-striving is the fifth attitude that includes you not forcing certain things to happen and letting everything happen as they should. In other words, you should try less for something in order to attain more. That may sound outrageous since life is all about striving and going after what we want, but the goal here is to be yourself and not change your values to achieve something. For example, we get stuck in the past by wondering "What if" or "If only I had tried harder". The problem with these thoughts is that everything that had happened is in the past and we live in the present. There is no point to strive to change what already happened. We should embrace our choices as well as the mistakes we have done and live in the present.

Acceptance is the sixth attitude of mindfulness and it urges us to accept things for what they are without trying to change them. Trying to deny things that have happened or are about to happen will stress you out. Whether it is a breakup or death, we have to come to terms with what has happened. Acceptance allows us to take the necessary measures for the future and helps us stay focused on reality. It helps us see what we truly want and enables us to do it in the present.

Letting go is the final attitude of mindfulness and it teaches us that letting go of ideas, people, behaviors, or anything that keeps us from living the present moment is good for us. We can't live our lives as they are in the present without letting go of the past or what holds us prisoners of enjoying every passing moment.

Mindfulness, like meditation, needs to be practiced daily, for as long as you are able to. There are many types of practices of mindfulness; some of them are Yin Yoga, Qigong, Mindful Eating, Body Scan Meditation, and Loving-Kindness Meditation. To start with, Yin Yoga is a type of yoga that includes slow paced sessions and the poses each person takes are maintained for longer than usual. This practice of mindfulness is stemming from the Taoist belief of yin and yang. Yang depicts a change, movement, and revelations while Yin represents the unmoving, stable, and hidden part. This concept can also be practiced on our bodies. The stiff connective tissues of your body, the ligaments, tendons, and fascia, are seen as yin and the mobile muscles including our blood are yang.

Yin Yoga is about the Yin parts of our body, the connective tissues which respond better to slow exercises. For example, if you maintain a yin pose for a certain amount of time, longer than usual, your body will take the cue to make them a little stronger as well as longer each time. For beginners, the recommended time to hold a pose is up to three minutes each and with practice, you will be able to maintain a pose for five minutes. Some recommended poses are the Reclined Cobbler's Pose or Supta Baddhakonasana, the Happy Baby Pose or Ananda Balasana, the Supine Twist or Jathara Parivrttanasana, the Thread-the-Needle Pose or Parsva Balasana, the Wide-Knee Child's Pose or Balasana, the Sphinx Pose or Salamba Bhujangasana, the Pigeon Pose or Raja Kapotasana, the Relaxation Pose or Savasana, and the Legs Up the Wall Pose or Viparita Karani.

When you change poses, you should be mindful and focused on your breath as well as the sensations your body has during each pose. If you find some poses to be difficult, don't give up on them, as we said before one of the attitudes of mindfulness is to be open to new experiences. As you move from one pose to the next, do it gently and be careful to never stretch to the point of inflicting any kind of pain to yourself. In each pose, you have to maintain stillness and surrender yourself to each position. Yin Yoga usually consists of passive poses that are held for a long time on the floor and help you exercise your pelvis, hips, inner thighs, and lower spine, areas that hold connective tissues.

Qigong is an extremely popular method of exercise in Chinese medicine and includes a combination of physical exercise and meditation. It is a method that promotes your health, your mental focus, and alleviates your stress. Also, it helps you maintain your Jing or what we call essence, the energy reserves of our bodies. With this method, you will have to harness your energy by allowing your twelve meridians to be open and accept the flowing energy. According to Chinese Medicine if one of your meridians is closed then there is a high chance of developing some kind of sickness in the area. The Twelve Meridians are:

o   Bright Yang Stomach Meridian of the Foot.
o   Greater Yin Spleen Meridian of the Foot.
o   Greater Yang Small Intestine Meridian of the Hand.
o   Lesser Yin Heart Meridian of the Hand.
o   Greater Yin Bladder Meridian of the Foot.
o   Lesser Yin Kidney Meridian of the Foot.
o   Faint Yin Pericardium Meridian of the Hand.
o   Lesser Yang Sanjiao Meridian of the Hand.
o   Lesser Yang Gallbladder Meridian of the Foot.

o   Faint Yin Lung Meridian of the Hand.

o   Bright Yang Large Intestine Meridian of the Hand.

o   Faint Yin Liver Meridian of the Foot.

Generally, scientists have admitted that Qigong helps in the relief of Arthritis, Cancer, Asthma, Chronic Fatigue, Headaches, Fibromyalgia, and many more. Qigong is separated into two parts, the internal Qigong and the external Qigong. The internal Qigong includes following a set of breathing exercises and meditation to achieve or maintain balance of yourself by using your energy to send it inside your body, resulting in enhancing its ability to heal and work properly. External Qigong is about using the energy you have harnessed in your body and apply it to someone else in order to heal him or her.

For beginners, it is recommended they start with MaBu or else the Horse Stance. This pose is used by many types of Asian martial arts and to start, you need to be in a wide position. Then, you must drop your hips down to the height of your knees while your back is still straight. Your ankles and your shin should be at a 90 degree angle and your knees should also be at a 90 degree angle with your shin and legs. Your feet should be 45 degrees outwards and your shoulders should be pulled back with your spine straight. Your head should face forward and your hands can be brought straight in front of you or you could bend your elbows behind your shoulders. This position should be held from ten to thirty seconds if this is your first time practicing it.

Another position that is recommended for beginners is Gongbu or else the Bow Stance that is also used often in Chinese martial arts. To practice Gongbu, you should place one foot forward and bend the knee of that leg slightly. The foot that is left behind should face 45 degrees outside and keep your back straight. Your one hand should face forward while the other should be bent to the elbow and place it to the side of your body. This pose should be held at first from ten to thirty seconds until you are able to do it for longer.

You could also practice Qigong sitting. Find a place to sit that makes you feel comfortable. Then, place your one palm up, to face the ceiling and have it close to your belly. The other palm should face downward and should be placed above your open palm. The two palms should have a considerable distance between each palm as if a ball was placed between them. When you feel ready, move around both your palms as if you were trying to sense this imaginary ball and feel the energy as your hands move. Your movements during all practice sessions of Qigong should be slow and gentle.

Mindful eating is a method that will help you control your eating habits and lessen binge eating. Through mindful eating, you will be able to reach a level of awareness of the subtle cues your body is sending you that has to do with eating such as hunger and cravings. You will acknowledge which food you really like or dislike and learn how to use all your senses when choosing which foods are healthier for your body. According to mindful eating, there is no wrong or right way to eat since everyone's eating methods and needs are special.

It is different from diets, especially popular ones since mindful eating is not focusing on restricting calories, but it gives us a choice to enhance the body's ability to control our eating habits. Eating because you will crave something, emotional eating, and binge eating will be able to control when you practice mindful eating since those are some of the reasons people usually gain weight and involve eating without control and mindlessly.

The first thing you can do when you are trying to practice mindful eating is to slow down the pace you eat. Since mindfulness promotes living in the moment, be aware of it and acknowledging the sensations and demands of your body, you should slow down and stop eating when your body signals you that it is full. For example, you could take short breaks between your bites and chew slowly. While you eat, your body and mind communicate so as to see if it is full. Your body sends its signals to your mind approximately twenty minutes after you start eating and this is often the reason why we end up overeating. However, if you eat at a slower pace, you will give your body and mind the time they need to communicate the necessary signals so as to stop or continue eating. You could chew each portion of food twenty-five times and you should always be seated when you eat. When we eat quickly, we don't let our body process the amount of food we eat and we don't give the chance it needs to signal that it is full.

It would also help if we didn't listen to our minds when it comes to food and focus on our body and whether or not it is indeed hungry. Is your stomach growling or you feel you are low on energy? Many times we eat because we are bored, lonely, sad, stressed or frustrated. Other times we eat during a movie or when we sit at our computers or in the car and not actually because we are hungry.

You should also develop a time schedule on when to eat. If you randomly eat meals at any time during the day, you may end up missing some and your hunger will make you eat way more than you should. This habit could affect your sleep and make our brain develop cues that are not entirely healthy for us. To achieve scheduling your meals, you could cook and store the meals for the next day beforehand. Also, when you eat along with friends or family it could be helpful since you will slow down to engage in conversation and actually enjoy your food.

Do not go shopping when you are hungry because you will end up buying unhealthy food that is quick to cook and eat. Added to this, you should think of where your food comes from and only see it as a product you buy from the market. Thinking about the process the food needed to pass in order for us to buy it and cook it, will make you more mindful of it and also bring you closer to nature. You will more thankful that you are able to eat such healthy foods and your body will thank you too. Take a moment to express your gratitude to everyone responsible for bringing this food to your plate and enjoy the opportunity you are given to enjoy it with your friends and family.

When you feel hungry, try to note how your hunger starts and when it ends. What foods make you full and which foods you need to eat more in order to satiate your hunger. Keep those things in mind for the next time you go shopping and which meals you should cook for the next day to eat. Eat only when you are genuinely hungry and try to savor the taste of your food because it may make you discover new flavors you will love to eat and be useful for your next trip to the market.

Also, try not to skip meals because your developing hunger will make it more difficult for you to be mindful when you are eating and it will lead you to eat anything when you are able to. Drinking water before you eat will help you eat the appropriate amount of food you need for your body and keep you from eating a larger portion of your meal than it is necessary. Most importantly be present when you eat and enjoy the moment. Don't think of anything else that can stress you and lead you to stress eating. Focus on the eating procedure and be thankful that you are able to eat this food that many people worked very hard for you to have on your plate.

Body scan meditation is a great way to connect you with your body and recognize the physical signs of stress and discomfort you may feel such as back or shoulder pain, headaches, and muscle tension and relieve them to an extent. Some people may have the signs and not even recognize they are stressed or troubled by a situation. This usually happens because they are not in an emotional state to accept the fact and also don't know how to read or ignore the signs their body sends them that it needs a break.

Body scan meditation will help you turn your focus on the parts of your body and the sensations associated with them while gradually shifting your attention from one part to the other, from your feet to your head. As you scan your body, you will be able to bring awareness to every single part of it and notice any subtle aches or tension associated with it. Your goal will be to acknowledge those cues and take the necessary measures to alleviate the problem after you are finished practicing body scan meditation. You should practice every day for as many times as you can, especially when you feel the need to do it.

To practice body scan meditation you should find a place to settle and sit that makes you comfortable to be able to relax your body as much as you can. You could also lay down since you will be scanning your whole body and many people practice body scan meditation before they fall asleep, but if you are not able to do so, sitting on the floor or on a chair will do just fine. Then, you should let your body get used to the position and the environment by taking a few deep and slow breaths and maintain this slow breathing pace for the rest of the session. Focus on breathing from your belly and try not to let your shoulders rise and fall with each breath you take.

Then, move your attention slowly to your feet and start noticing the sensations on them. Are you noticing any pain? Acknowledge it as well as any emotions that go with that pain. Focus on those sensations that cause you discomfort and imagine the tension separating from your body through each breath you take and then vanish into thin air. Stay there for a few seconds after you have acknowledged those sensations visualized them leaving your body and move on to the next part when you feel ready.

Continue the same pattern with every area of your body, as you will gradually move up until you reach your head. If you feel any discomfort, pain or pressure, take deep breaths and imagine those uncomfortable sensations leave your body. When you are finished, you will feel the tension leave your body and as you keep practicing you will also be more aware of your body and any possible subtle pain or tension that may accumulate in the future. You can practice body scan meditation any time you feel stressed even if it is for more than one time each day.

Another part of being mindful and practicing mindfulness it the loving-kindness meditation method that is part of self-care and will help you enhance your abilities to forgive others and accept yourself for what it is, that includes your body too. When you practice love-kindness meditation, you will focus your pure, loving, and fair energy to yourself and to other people. You will experience some warm feelings of compassion and realize why loving yourself and others is so important for everyone to do so.

During the session of loving-kindness meditation, you will have to pick certain targets, including yourself, to aim with your loving energy. Pick any quiet time during the day you may have, even on your breaks at work, and try to make yourself comfortable in a seated position. Then, close your eyes and try to relax your body by taking a few deep and slow breaths. Visualize yourself feeling the effects of emotional and physical wellness as well as inner calmness. Imagine the love you feel for yourself, acknowledge it, and let it grow.

Take the time to thank yourself for what you have accomplished so far, no matter how small, and accept the fact that you are alright the way you are now. As you visualize those things, keep in mind that as you breathe in, you take inside yourself love and breathe out the tension you may have. If you find your thoughts being interrupted, redirect your attention back to the feeling of calmness and immense love. Let those feelings engulf you and become lost in them. Then, you can have a choice to stay lost in those loving thoughts or redirect your focus to your loved ones and experience the love and gratefulness you feel towards them.

When you are finished with your meditation, open your eyes and relish in the lingering sensations of this wonderful experience. You can repeat this session any time you want during the day and anytime you feel stressed or the need to feel loved and appreciated.

If you don't want to choose a particular mindfulness meditation type, you also have the choice to practice the basic mindfulness meditation method that will help you develop mindfulness and be mindful about each moment of your life. You should start by finding a quiet place that makes you feel comfortable and sit on the floor or on a chair. You need to have your back and neck straight but be careful not to be stiff. You should also wear clothes that make you comfortable to avoid distractions.

Set aside all thoughts that are linked to your past and to the future to allow your mind to focus on the present moment. Focus and become aware of your breath and feel the sensation of the air moving in, out, and around your body. Pay attention to every thought that comes and passes, even those that include anxiety, fear, or worry. It is important not to ignore them. If your mind wanders off to other things, observe the direction they are headed to and without judging yourself for this outcome, bring your thoughts back to the present moment and sensations. When you are finished with your session, sit still for a minute or more if you feel the need to, and be aware of the place you are at before getting up.

Being mindful is an important skill to enjoy the present moments we come across since most people do not appreciate them or live them to the fullest until they become a pleasant or unpleasant memory. However, keep in mind that moments come and go, but your body will always be with you and this is why it is extremely important to be mindful about your body too. As you practice mindfulness of any type, you can add to the session ways of being mindful of your body too.

For example, as you sit on the floor or on a chair in an upright posture you could turn your focus on the sensation of your whole body. Sense the contact of the floor or chair on your body and how it feels, sense how the clothes feel on your skin and how the air impacts your body.

You could also turn your focus on the parts of your body that feel tight or relaxed, cold or heated, and so on. You can focus entirely on pleasant or unpleasant sensations of your body to relish in them or fix them.

If you practice mindfulness of the body in different places, notice how your body reacts in each location and after certain changes. When you are finished with your session try to stay focused on how your body feels during different situations you will encounter during the rest of your day.

Following the different types of mindfulness meditation will impact your life and the way you see the world in a great and pleasant manner. When you start seeing the results of connecting to your body and to your mind or actually letting them work together as it happens in mindful eating, you will be the witness of a change to a healthier lifestyle. There are several more methods that are able to nurture your connection to your body and train you in how to listen to it such as Chakra meditation and Somatic meditation both of which we will analyze in later chapters.

Chapter 4: How to Listen to Your Body: Chakra Meditation

The Vedas are the oldest written scripts in India, which originate from 1.500 to 500 B.C and are recorded from the oral tradition of the upper class Brahmins. Form there we learn of the chakra system that was then spelled as chakra. At first, the meaning of the word chakra was "wheel", referring to the chariot wheels of the ruler that were called Chakravartins of that time and it was also used as a metaphor for the sun. There were some mentions of the chakras as they exist today in the Yoga Upanishads of the 600 B.C and in Yoga Sutras of Patanjali of 200 B.C.

The chakra system rose along with Kundalini Yoga inside the Tantric Tradition. The word Tantra is translated as a tool (tra) for stretching (tan). But what is chakra? Chakras are concentrated energy in our bodies; they are spinning "wheels" of energy. Humans have major and minor chakras and when most people talk about chakras they mean the main seven physical ones that we will analyze shortly. Each of the chakras we have in our body connects us to the Universal Life Force Energy of the Universe. The system of Chakras is essential for the energy to flow from the Universe right into our bodies. Aside from the seven main Chakras, we have twenty-one minor chakras all over the body which are grouped under ten bilateral minor chakras that are found to the hand, elbow, foot, navel, ear, shoulder, and clavicles.

Chakra meditation is essential for people who want to learn how to listen to their bodies since if we do not provide the necessary support to them with the right food and vitamins then we will have less energy in the body. On the other hand, when we take care of our bodies through physical means and mental exercises we will have enough energy to be as productive as we wish. Chakra meditation helps you with energy flow and feeling more energized than ever. What are the locations of the chakras and what are their characteristics?

We will start with the first chakra that is named Root Chakra or Muladhara, which stems from the words Mula that means root and Dhara which means support. The role of this chakra is to ground you with the earth, in other words, to connect your energy with the earth. The Root Chakra is located at the base of your spine and more specifically near your tailbone and it ends bellow your belly button. It controls your basic survival needs and when energy flows through this Chakra you are able to feel secure as well as confident that you are able to satisfy your needs. It is the Root Chakra's role to provide you with all the tools you need to survive such as emotional security. The color representing the Root Chakra is red and when it is balanced you will be connected to the full experience of being human.

When the Root Chakra is overactive, you will be anxious and jittery because you will feel afraid. Fear is used and linked to the natural need we have to survive, to be alive. For example, you may have a successful job that makes you financially secure, but you will be constantly afraid of the possibility of losing this job and your financial security when the Root Chakra is overactive. It will give your mind subtle cues of the need to survive, even when you do not face any real threat. On a physical level, you may feel lower back pain, problems digesting food or hip pain.

In the case where your survival needs are generally being met, then the Root Chakra may become underactive. This could lead you to daydream or feel less connected to reality and more connected to what could have been different in your life, to your dreams. This may not seem as a bad situation, but being balanced is extremely important to keep your basic needs under control. For example, if you are in a constant state of daydreaming, you may neglect your present needs and end up with an overactive Root Chakra.

The law of Karma rules the Root Chakra which means that each action you take will result in an equal reaction. To make sure that your actions have positive reactions, you can put your body to good use and determine the possible endgame of your choices. In other words, you should listen to the cues your body sends you since the Root Chakra is all about fulfilling your basic needs. Your body will feel either comfortable or uncomfortable when you are about to make a choice and evaluates the threat level corresponding to those decisions.

To balance your Root Chakra, except from chakra meditation we will analyze shortly, you need to engage in physical exercise, you need to give the necessary nutrition to your body by eating red fruits, and connect to the earth by gardening, walking barefoot in nature or start swimming. You could also take baths with essential oils such as Rosewood, Sandalwood, Cedar, Ginger or Rosemary for relaxation.

The second chakra is named Sacral Chakra or else Svadhishana which means "the place of the self". The Sacral Chakra is about the identity of one's self and whatever he or she chooses to do with it. Out of all the chakras, this is the one who has to do with creativity and all the forms a person can express it since it is responsible for bringing you creative energy. It is related to your emotions, so it is the one who enables you to enjoy every moment you live as well as your successes in every aspect of your life. The color associated with the Sacral Chakra is orange and is located below your belly button and reaches its center.

When your second chakra is balanced, you will be able to enjoy everything life will throw your way from relationships, good food to sexuality and creative activities without overdoing it. However, if balance is not achieved and your second chakra is overactive you will face problems such as addictions or excess eating that will lead you to feel guilty for enjoying things that were ought to make you feel good because those things will not be healthy anymore. They may lead to obesity or restlessness and guilty emotions that will prevent you from being yourself and express your creativity and emotions in a healthy way.

On the other hand, if your Sacral Chakra is underactive by your focusing on every detail of everything and not enjoy or be thankful for each moment you are able to live or not give yourself enough credit for everything you have accomplished, you may get depressed and feel as if you are not enough for anyone or as if everything you do will never be enough to succeed. You will lack inspiration and creativity, symptoms that will be harmful to your body and spirit. You can balance your second chakra by wondering if your choices are good for you and healthy.

Think about the consequences of your actions and let your body and mind guide you in the right direction. Emotions are an integral part of our choices, but sometimes we have to listen to our mind and body to choose the appropriate path for us. Enjoy life, eat healthily, and maintain healthy relationships. This way you will be able to energize your Sacral Chakra.

The third chakra is named Solar Plexus or else Manipura in Sanskrit which means "lustrous gem". The Solar Plexus is responsible for your identity, power, self-confidence, expression of your will, and mental abilities. There must be times when you found yourself in situations that you knew instinctively how right or wrong they were for you by some cues your body was sending you. Most people would call it gut feeling, but this is the power of your Solar Plexus when it reacts. It makes you feel physically confident about a situation you are in. The color associated with the third chakra is yellow and is located at the center of your belly button and reaches the upper part of your belly. When the third chakra is balanced, you will get a feeling of continues wisdom where you will know almost all the time what is right or wrong for you. You will be decisive and empowered to act as you deem appropriate without ever doubting yourself.

On the other hand, when the Solar Plexus is not balanced and overactive when the power you have over your life transfers into the lives of other people, you may get angry quickly before even thinking about the reasons that got you angry in the first place. You will feel the need to control every little detail of your life and the life of others, lacking a key element in your every day encounters and that is empathy and also, the ability to feel compassion towards others.

You will become manipulative and misuse the power you may have over others. When the third chakra is underactive, you will lose all the power you exercised over yourself and probably be depended on others, you may also feel insecure, you wouldn't have the power anymore to make decisions and confidence will give way to neediness. You will lack having a purpose in life and a sense of direction. You can fix all that by focusing on the things that you are good at. By focusing on your abilities and skills, you will build up your confidence again in order to feel empowered once more.

The Solar Plexus chakra is all about expressing yourself, your abilities both physical and intellectual, personal power, and your motivation to turn your dreams into reality. If you find that you lack in those aspects, make a list of everything that represents you and everything you excelled before this situation brought you down. Remember everything you had accomplished and make them happen once again.

The fourth chakra is your Heart or else Anahata Chakra which means in Sanskrit "unhurt". Since it is located on your chest area which includes your heart, Anahata Chakra is responsible for your feelings of love, compassion, and bringing color and beauty to your life. It is often referred to as the bridge that brings together your physical body with your spirituality because it is located exactly in the middle of the seven chakras and connects the lower chakras which are referred to as the physical world and the higher chakras which are the spiritual world. The Heart Chakra is also associated with the love yourself and the love you are capable to feel for other people as well as the world around you including animals and nature. Your kindness also stems from the fourth chakra too and can control the intensity of these emotions. The color associated with the Heart Chakra is green and when it is balanced you will be able to feel love equally for both yourself and the others, even when you will go through tough times.

At the times when the heart chakra is overactive, you will lose the boundaries you have set for yourself and start making choices that are not healthy for you all because of love. For example, you will place the needs of others ahead of yours and you will end up losing your self-worth and your needs will be unmet for long periods of time, something that will definitely be not healthy for you. Keep in mind that it is essential to treat yourself with the same amounts of love and kindness you give to others.

On the other hand, when your fourth chakra is underactive you will become distant from other people since you will feel as if it is really hard to get close and form a connection with anyone. This happens due to the fact that life tends to throw in our way a lot of heartbreak and at some point, you will have to deal with betrayal. Those moments should be faced as a teaching moment and keep the lessons of those situations close as to not repeat the same mistakes we did to the past.

However, it can be hard for most people not to take the results and pain of heartbreak personally for longer than necessary. You may even feel the need to build a wall around your emotions and forbid yourself from letting anyone get close to your heart because you will feel afraid of the past repeating itself. You may also feel as if you can't connect with your body and find it difficult to communicate your emotional needs with your physical needs.

To bring balance to your Heart Chakra, you need to start by bringing love back into your life. You could even take back some of the love you give to others when your fourth chakra is overactive or bring down the walls you have built around your heart and let people get close to you again. Most of all treat yourself right by appreciating you and remember everything you have been through as a lesson you had to be taught. When you are able to love yourself again, then you will succeed in letting people love you and return that love in a healthy way so as to not neglect your own needs. The key is in how you see yourself. If you love your appearance and personality, others will love them too.

What you need to keep in mind that your Heart Chakra is all about love for yourself and others, relationships, acceptance and compassion, change and forgiveness, and your ability to grieve and move on. Once you have mastered all those things through meditation and mindfulness, your mind and body will be open for you to read as easy as you breathe. The fifth chakra is the Throat Chakra or else the Vishuddha which means "pure". As the name of the fifth chakra suggests it is located at the center of the neck and that includes the throat. It works as a passage through which flows the energy between the lower chakras and the head. The Throat Chakra enables people to express themselves and communicate effectively. It gives voice to a person's truth and thoughts. The energy to speak comes from the fifth chakra on a spiritual level since we all know how we are able to speak on a physical level.

The color associated with the fifth chakra is blue and when it is balanced you will be able to speak out what you believe clearly along with love and kindness. You will know the exact words you will need to speak for each situation you will find yourself in. Those around you will be inspired by your ability to know exactly what to say and by your kind and wise words.

However, your Throat Chakra may be overactive when you have tried for a long time to make your voice heard to the people that are close to you. You may have felt ignored for long or that others dismiss your opinions too often and you have tried to tackle this problem by speaking more intensely and louder. If that is the case and your fifth chakra is overactive, you will notice that you interrupt other people often when they speak and people may tell you that you love to listen to yourself speak since you will talk more than it is necessary to make your point. On a physical level, you may have symptoms of throat pain or persistent infections.

On the other hand, when your fifth chakra is underactive, you will never speak the truth you believe in and refuse to speak up. People may think you a quiet person by nature or shy and often you will find yourself unable to describe your emotions or find it difficult to find the courage needed to talk back to someone. An underactive fifth chakra occurs for the same reasons as an overactive chakra. You have been ignored and dismissed for too long. You can balance your Throat Chakra by thinking before you speak, especially about serious matters. For example, think if your words you are going to utter are true or necessary. Are they kind or they are intended to hurt someone? Practice describing your emotions out loud even if no one is around to hear you. It doesn't matter if people are not around, sometimes when we voice our emotions it is easier for us to accept them and acknowledge their existence.

An imbalanced Throat Chakra will result in you not being able to control the things you say and you will not be able to listen and understand what other people are talking about. You will be afraid of speaking to everyone including yourself, and even if you speak, your voice will be heard as small and insignificant. You may also end up telling lies to avoid analyzing a matter you have to discuss with someone and you will not be able to keep secrets or hold your word.

The fifth chakra helps you to express yourself, to be able to speak out and to communicate with others and with yourself. As important it is to listen to your body, it is equally important to listen to your emotions and let them connect with your physical presence in the world. Being in tune with your emotions as well as your body will make your life much easier and open up many more paths for you to solve any problem that may come your way.

The sixth chakra is called The Third Eye Chakra or Ajna which means "perceiving". It is located on the forehead and between the eyebrows; therefore it is used for intuition and foresight. The color associated with The Third Eye Chakra is indigo and is often associated with the pineal gland located in the brain and regulates the time you sleep as well as the time you wake up. The Third Eye Chakra is responsible for your vision, intuition, receiving information beyond the five senses that is often perceived as a psychic ability, it connects you to wisdom and insight, and it motivates creativity and inspiration in you.

When The Third Eye Chakra is balanced, you will be in tune with both the material and the spiritual world and it is very difficult for the sixth chakra to be overactive. However, when an occasion such as an overactive sixth chakra occurs, you will find yourself focused on psychic activities such as astrology, tarot cards, and paranormal occurrences. These activities will overwhelm you and keep you from experiencing and enjoying your everyday life. When your sixth chakra is underactive, which is more common, you will feel disconnected from activities that enhance your spiritual presence such as meditation that is needed to balance your Third Eye Chakra.

Generally, imbalance of your sixth chakra includes feelings of being stuck in the daily routine and not being able to see beyond your problems creating a dead end for moving on, not being able to make your dreams come true, and it will make your reject anything spiritual or beyond what we have used to believe in. You will be dismissive that there is more in life than having a routine to stick to and feel safe in. You will not be able to connect to nature or to your emotions as well as your body.

The seventh and final chakra is named The Crown Chakra or else Sahaswara which means "a thousand petals". It is located at the top of our head and is enables us to access higher levels of consciousness as we realize that there is more in life than personal prejudices. A person's consciousness is located in the seventh chakra, but it is more connected to the energy of the universe than with ours. The color of the seventh chakra is often white or deep purple. The Crown Chakra connects your energy with the rest of the universe and the task of balancing it is the goal of the Buddhist concept of reaching nirvana. The moment you achieve the balance of The Crown Chakra you have beaten pain and death.

A balanced Crown Chakra offers you pure consciousness, wisdom or acknowledgment of everything that is sacred. It connects you with the limitless energy and possibilities provided by the universe and liberate you from any limitations of the physical world. Last but not least, it offers you pure bliss and spiritual ecstasy. An imbalanced Crown Chakra can be seen as being completely out of tune with your spirit and express continues cynicism and condensation to everything that is sacred or even be completely disconnected from your body. This may result in finding solace and meaning to fantasies and dreams inside your head that will make you distant from reality and the present moment.

Meditation will help you open all your chakras and especially the first six since The Crown Chakra is not that easy to balance or energize. However, if you manage to balance all the other six chakras, you will not have to endure the consequences of an imbalanced seventh chakra. Except for meditation, you could also try using chakra stones which when you interact with will affect both your physical and mental health. The stones for each chakra are the following.

1. The Root Chakra: Smokey Quartz, Hematite, and Black Onyx.
2. The Sacral Chakra: Sunstone and Tigers' Eye.
3. The Solar Plexus Chakra: Pyrite and Jasper.
4. The Heart Chakra: Aventurine and Rose Quartz.
5. The Throat Chakra: Sodalite and Aquamarine.
6. The Third Eye Chakra: Lolite, Amethyst, and Fluorite.
7. The Crown Chakra: Moonstone, Clear Quartz, and Amethyst.

Now that we have analyzed the basics concerning the seven chakras that exist in our bodies, it is time to present how meditation will help you open up your chakras and as a result make you feel more energized and in tune with your emotions and body. The first step to chakra meditation is to find a quiet place and sit on the floor or on a chair still for a few moments while taking deep breaths. This way, you will leave the stress and tension behind you. This is the moment when you get in tune with your body and how it feels at the present.

When you feel in tune with your body and the sensations it gives off, bring your focus on the base of your spine and imagine a spinning, bright red light. Feel it move at the same time as you breathe and stand there for a moment with your focus drawn on it.

Then, move your attention slowly up your spine and let it rest on the area below your belly button. There, you will witness a bright, warm, spinning orange light that is in tune with your breath too. You should also stay at this are for a few moments until you feel comfortable with it.

When you finish, move your attention slowly up to the area above your belly button. As you focus all your attention on this area, you will feel strong emotions radiating from it such as love, fear or calmness. You will witness a bright, warm and spinning yellow light and again, you should pause for a moment until you get comfortable in its presence. Then, move your attention up to your chest area and more specifically, to where your heart is. There, you will encounter a bright green spinning light. As you focus and connect with it, you may feel the need to place your hand above the spot where your heart is. Don't hesitate to do so, it will help you connect with the area more.

The moment you are finished, move again your attention up and to your throat. There, you will imagine the existence of a bright blue light that spins. In this area, you might feel the need to clear your throat or swallow. Don't try to stop yourself from doing that since it will be a natural response to turning your whole attention there, especially if you practice chakra meditation for the first time.

Then, move your focus to the space between your eyebrows where your third eye rests. You will encounter a bright, deep indigo light. The light also spins and will become brighter with each passing second. When you are done getting used to and connect with your third eye chakra move to the final chakra that rests at the top of your head. There, you will see a spinning violet or white light that is very bright. This is the light that connects you to the universe and therefore as you focus on it, you will feel at peace and a sense of calmness that may blow you away. When you are done connection and being comfortable with the final chakra, take a deep breath and when you feel ready to open your eyes. Don't rise instantly, but take a moment to acknowledge your surroundings and get used to returning to the present moment.

Learning about the seven chakras and their meaning to our lives will help you get more in tune with your emotions, mind, and body. Everything in the universe consists of energy and we are not the exception. The process and success of listening to our bodies do not only include getting physical exercise and eating healthy but also includes our efforts to listen to every subtle cue it may send us through meditation and mindfulness.

Chapter 5: How to Listen to Your Body: Somatic Mindfulness and Kundalini Meditation

By now, you may think that listening to your body is an extremely difficult process or even that you have no need to practice everything that was mentioned before because you already know everything there is to know about your body's cues to you. That may be true, but there are always things gone unnoticed by man people when it comes to their bodies. For example, there is one of the most basic responses our body possesses that we do not know how it works exactly and all of us have experienced. The flight-or-fight response.

The flight-or-fight response or else the acute stress response is a psychological reaction that happens when we are in the presence of something that is terrifying to us either mentally or physically. When this response happens, hormones are released throughout our body to prepare us to deal with the threat or run towards a safe place. The name of this phenomenon derives from our ancestors during the ancient times who would either stay and face any threat that came their way or flee. No matter the choice we make, our body prepares us to face the incoming danger.

When we endure extreme levels of stress, our nervous system is put into action because there is a sudden release of hormones. The adrenal glands are stimulated by the sympathetic nervous system and the distribution of catechol amines is triggered, which include both noradrenaline and adrenaline. The results of this occurrence are increased heart rate, breathing rate, and blood pressure. When the danger has passed, it will take between twenty and sixty minutes for our bodies to return back to normal.

Another sign of flight-or-fight response it flushed or pale skin. As the stress starts to get a grip on you, the blood flow to the surface of the body is reduced to start flowing to the brain, legs, arms, and muscles. This will result in you getting pale or to your face being flushed as blood will rush to your brain and head. Your pupils will dilate since the body will also prepare you to be more observant and aware of your surroundings during the time you will have to face a threat. So, dilated pupils will offer you a better vision. Last but not least, you may also sense yourself trembling since your muscles will become more tense and ready to take action.

The above was only one example of how our body works even in dangerous situations that we may not even know what kind of response we are having or why we are acting a certain way. Being in tune with our bodies and knowing how to connect with them is a necessary skill to develop and the process of doing so will help you find out more things about yourself that haven't paid any attention to. So, it is not always true that we know everything there is to learn about our bodies. To this journey, an important method we could use is Somatic Mindfulness.

Somatic Mindfulness will help us build a connection between our mind and body, especially in the areas that there was no connection. It enables us to use the responses of our body as a source of information about our current state and our emotions. It comes as no surprise that Somatic Mindfulness is used as a way to cure emotional traumas since it can be utilized as a way to enhance our ability to regulate the nervous system by helping us release the emotions we may have help inside us unconsciously and feel them in a physical level.

Somatic Meditation is met in Tibetan and East Asian Buddhism as well as in spiritual Taoism. As the name suggests, in Somatic Meditation the main tool used is the body and in a lesser amount, the mind. The concept behind Somatic Mindfulness is that your spirit, mind, body, and emotions are all connected together. When you practice Somatic Meditation, you will feel less stressed, less pain, less anger or frustration, and it will help you get over past traumatic events. Essentially you will be free of all the things that are preventing you from listening to your body and live a healthy life.

However, you should be aware that when you practice Somatic Meditation overwhelming and painful emotions of a past trauma will come back to you in order for you to deal with them. Don't be surprised or try to end the session because a past emotional heartbreak or shock will have to be dealt with eventually and through Somatic Meditation, you will be able to deal with this occurrence in a controlled way.

When you start your sessions of Somatic Mindfulness, try exercising for at least once a week for a two month period, even though it is recommended for you to practice more than once a week. But if you wish to practice other forms of meditation at the same time, you can opt for a once a week session of Somatic Meditation. After you have finished practicing each time, give yourself a minute or two before you start any type of interaction with other people. You need time to fully acknowledge and take in the experience you just finished doing because sensing your body this way for the first time will be a powerful experience. For example, you will need to ask yourself how you feel after the session is over, has anything changed in the way you hold yourself? Do you feel any different? When you answer these questions, you can open your eyes and focus on the room you are in for a few moments to focus on your new feelings and take in your surroundings, on how you see the world now. Is it different?

Before you start practicing, stand up and ponder on how you feel at the moment before you begin your exercises. Focus on how your breathing is and pinpoint the location of where you have focused your attention and energy. For example, how does your energy feel when you focus on it? Do you feel calm and serene or do you sense negative emotions and by extent energy that makes you unsettled and fidgety? What do you need to heal? If you don't feel anything there is no need to worry or give up thinking that you are fine. Those emotions may reveal themselves to you later and if they don't, then continue because Somatic Mindfulness will help you connect on a deeper level your mind with your body, spirit, and emotions.

The exercises start with grounding. Stand up and let your eyes not focus on anything. Watch the room without actually seeing it. Then, raise yourself slowly on your toes and drop down to your heels. Keep up this exercise in a slow rhythm while at the same time thinking that all your weight drops through your heels. Keep this exercise up for a minute or until you feel the jolts of your hips and lower back loosen considerably.

After you have finished with the first part of this practice, take a short break but do not break the position you are in now. Then, create a small bouncing in your legs by using your knees and letting them bend slightly. Turn into a straight position by pushing backwards again and softly shake your legs. Focus and imagine that his soft shaking rocks your whole body and moves through your hips, up to your shoulders and reaches your neck. Let this exercise relax your jaw, your tail bone, and lower back until the duration of one minute passes.

Once your jaw, tail bone, and lower back are relaxed, take a short break and bring yourself back to a standing position. Let your hands rest at the front of your thighs while you start focusing on your breath. Inhale slowly and as you do that bring your chin forward and softly move your hips backward. Then, move your upper body forward so that you have created an arch with your back. Stay in this position for a moment, for around eight breaths, and later, as you continue breathing slowly, let your head fall relaxed down. Then, move your tail bone under and forward, around your back until you bring yourself into the position you were when you started. During this exercise, your focus should be on your breaths and your spine, on how it moves.

When the above exercise is over, resume your standing position and slowly sway back and forth as a bamboo does when hit by a soft gust of wind. You will feel all the accumulated tension leave your body. If you happen to feel little tremors on your body, don't try to stop them. This is the way your body releases tension.

In the end, stay still for a moment and focus on the sensations you have inside and are finally able to notice now. Can you feel more relaxed and less tense? Do you feel any different your feet and legs? More charged with energy perhaps? More alive?

Let us take a look at another type of exercise. Start by standing and letting your eyes look but focus on nothing. Place one leg forward by putting down your heel first and later your whole foot on the ground. Then, shift your weight forward and on that front foot without letting your back foot leave the ground. As you step forward, reach out with the same arm as your forward foot, with fingers outstretched. When your foot is on the floor, close your hand as though you grabbed something and don't forget to breathe all the while. When you reached this position, one foot forward and a hand turned into a fist, pause for a while and then, bring yourself into a standing position by setting your foot next to the other, by releasing your grip and letting your hand loose on your side. Do this exercise for two minutes on one side and two minutes on the other side. During this practice, keep your focus on your hand, foot, and breaths.

When you have finished with all sides, don't move and stay in a standing position. You may start feeling the sway from the exercise starting on its own. Don't try to stop it, but go with the flow all the while checking on how you feel. Does your body feel any different?

One last type of exercise, we are going to mention here is the following. Start by bringing yourself in a standing position and focus on your breath. Then, take a deep inhale and as you let this breath go, make a shhh sound with your mouth. Imagine you are telling to someone to keep quiet. You can even make the sound if you want to. As you do it, focus on how it makes you feel, especially on the area that covers your chest and your stomach. This sound should last until your breath is finished and then take another deep inhale and repeat the process. Keep in mind that this should be done for approximately eight breaths. The shhh sound is extremely useful for the opening of the diaphragm which sometimes is tight on occasions such as being afraid.

Next, inhale again deeply, and now utter the sound mmm, as you let your breath out. Press your lips together and find the appropriate pressure that will create the most vibration for your whole head. Keep making the sound for as long as you can keep up and then repeat the inhale process for around eight breaths. You should shift your focus on the vibrations caused by the sound that can be felt in your head. The humming sound can stimulate the vagus nerve which is the main branch of the parasympathetic nervous system. This way we will be able to relax by resetting the over-aroused nervous system.

When you are finished with this exercise, stand still and straight for a minute and check the sensations of your body as well as your emotions that may be new and noticed now. Do you feel any shudders or swaying movement? Do you feel the need to stretch? Don't try to stop it or avoid it, do what your body wants and move along with it. Do you feel any different than before you started this exercise? Maybe you noticed a difference in your breathing or any change in your sense of space? Maybe now you are able to put words on those sensations you experienced.

As we were able to see, Somatic Meditation is centered on the body and seeks to develop the connection of your body and mind as well as your connection to them. So, pay attention to your physical responses during the session of you practicing Somatic Meditation and with practice, you will be able to see more results. Awakening your body will have a profound effect on how you view yourself and will make you appreciate your body more than you already do.

One last method we will analyze that will help you start listening to your body more effectively is Kundalini which is a Sanskrit term which means primal energy and is coming from ancient India to teach us about a form of energy that has been roped at the base of our spine from the moment we were born and is also the source of our life force. Kundalini may be freed from the base of our spine by spiritual practices. Kundalini meditation helps you channel your energy and release all the stress that exists in your body.

Kundalini meditation is a part of Kundalini yoga and its goal is to move energy throughout your body starting from your root chakra located at the spine. This energy that is placed there has to be set free and go through all the seven chakras that exist in our bodies and then leave through the crown chakra that is placed above our heads. When we release energy from our body through this process, we create a communication path for the mind and the body to tackle physical, spiritual, and mental problems.

To practice Kundalini Meditation, the first thing you need to do is finding a location that makes you feel at peace and where no one is going to interrupt you. Keep in mind that the best time to practice is in the morning as soon as you wake up because the chances of being bothered are less. Another appropriate time for you to practice is at night, right before you go to sleep so as to destress and recuperate after a tiring day. Bring a bottle of water with you and choose clean, comfortable, and fresh clothes that will not bother you during your practice. Before you start, set a timeframe of how long would you like to practice, it could vary from a few minutes to a few hours. However, for beginners, it would be recommended a length of eleven minutes.

Take a seat on the floor with your legs crossed or even sit on a chair but place your weight on your feet. If you want to be even more comfortable when you are on the floor, you can choose to sit on a pillow or a cotton blanket. In both positions, your back should be straight. Then, lower your eyes slowly until they are approximately 90% closed. Regulate your breaths and chant a mantra to focus. A good choice for beginners is the mantra "Sat Nam" which means "truth is my identity" and it helps you direct your energy. Say "Sat" as you inhale and "Nam" as you exhale and as you do this, focus on the words you say out loud or imagine them being written in your head. This mantra can be also used during stressful situations you have on any day. You will have your own mantra that signals your breaking away from an old state and reflect on the state you want to be at the exact moment you chant it.

Kundalini meditation will help you let the everyday stress you may get from a hectic work environment or from problems you may currently face, go and turn it into peace. It will also teach you the right way to breathe and open up the capacity of your lungs. Added to this, you will be able to concentrate in an easier way than you did before and any random thoughts you may have will be prevented so as to not disturb your balance. You will learn how to be aware of your body and connect it with your mind and your spirit.

It is believed that Kundalini meditation can also help people who suffer from various addictions, depression, phobias, fatigue, grief, anxiety, obsession, sleep disorders such as insomnia, learning disorders, compulsions, and stress. It is important for you to not give up on practicing even though it may seem hard at first. All you need is more time and practice to be able to reach a level where you will be satisfied.

We live in a world where we come face to face with constant change, even we change many times during our life and we may not even notice it. Practicing meditation in all its types and forms will let you tackle those changes in the best way possible, not to mention you will be able to identify the changing needs of your body. Imagine what it would feel like to notice any subtle change your body goes through, to know the signals of almost every need of your body. It would save us a lot of time and pain from searching what is happening inside us.

However, to take care of your body, you need to know how to develop an emotional resilience and constantly work on it. An essential part of self-care is developing the necessary skills to be prepared and face any stressful situation whether it is something serious or something light.

Chapter 6: Develop Your Emotional Resilience

Emotional resilience is the ability to handle stressful situations. The more resilient is someone, the more he is able to adapt to change without having any lasting difficulties. However, people who are less resilient don't handle as well as they should the stress and many changes they could come across their lives whether they are minor or major. Experts say that people who can handle minor stress reason in an easier way, they can also deal with major stress crises in an effective way. So, we can conclude from the start that resilience has many benefits for our everyday survival and state of mind.

Before we start analyzing the matter of resilience and how we could develop emotional resilience, we should understand what exactly we are talking about when we say stress since this is a word we have mentioned numerous times throughout the course of this book. Stress is what happens when we face a threat or a major challenge in our lives and that triggers a specific biological response during which hormones and chemicals are released throughout our body. Stress is the very thing that triggers our fight-or-flight response because the body needs to either fight the very thing that stresses us out or run away from it.

If we see it from the above perspective, stress is not necessarily a bad thing; it helps us when we are threatened. Stress is the very thing that helped our ancestors survive and it can help us today to avoid dangerous situations such as meeting our project's deadline, make us react quickly when we come face to face with having an accident or help you keep calm whenever others are throwing a tantrum. The stressors, things that trigger the stress response vary from people to people and may not even share the same attributes. For example, many people like speaking in public, but others hate it and each one has his or her own reason for doing so.

Stress isn't always bad, but the cases of it having severe consequences is when people are exposed to it for a prolonged period of time and can both physically and mentally hurt those people who are exposed for so long to it. If you consider the fact that when people are exposed to frequent adrenaline surges can lead them to damaged blood vessels, higher risks of heart attack and stroke, anxiety, headaches, insomnia, weight gain, and high blood pressure, then stress is not a healthy condition to have for the rest of your life. Three types of stress are acute stress, episodic acute stress, and chronic stress among other types.

Acute stress is what usually happens to everyone. The body reacts immediately to a situation that is a challenge or a threat to someone. For example, this is what people experience when they escape from a car accident. It may also be the frightening and yet exciting feeling of riding a roller coaster or when you bungee jump. These occurrences of acute stress don't hurt your health under normal circumstances. It is believed that these situations may even help you since they practice your brain in developing the appropriate response to possible future stressful situations. However, there is also severe acute stress that will be extremely harmful to your health and this is what you get when faced with a situation that will threaten your life and can lead you to develop post-traumatic stress disorder.

Episodic acute stress happens when you encounter persistent episodes of acute stress. This is the case when you are anxious about things that are about to happen or that you suspect they may happen. You may be unsatisfied with your life and think of it as chaotic with you jumping from one problem to the next and that is causing you recurring acute stress episodes. People, who work in professions such as police officers or firefighters that have to deal with high-stress situations, have such episodes. As it happens with severe acute stress, episodic acute stress can also take a toll on your mental and physical health.

Chronic stress is what happens when you are exposed to high levels of stress for a long period of time. It suffices to say that being stressed for such a long period of time, your health will suffer. More specifically you endanger yourself to developing depression, anxiety, cardiovascular disease, weakened immune system, or high blood pressure. You will also have to endure headaches, difficulty when trying to sleep, and an upset stomach.

It is a fact that stress can make it extremely difficult for a person to control his or her emotions even when they are facing mild cases of stress. Their personal relationships may suffer from expressing their frustration as well as their work is possible to suffer too. Stress is also linked to diseases such as lung disease and fatal accidents. Children that are suffering from chronic stress are more prone to developing mental illnesses if this condition is not treated appropriately.

Stress can also lead to premature aging and it weakens your immune system. High stress levels place a toll on the immune system, which in results makes you more exposed to catching a cold and have infections. The causes of stress are too many and vary from person to person. Some common examples can be living through a chronic illness, being the victim of a crime, having gone through an abusive relationship or an unhappy marriage, living in poverty or being homeless, and working in a dangerous profession.

When you are stressed, you may experience symptoms such as insomnia and other sleep related problems, chronic pain, losing your appetite or eating too much, having concentration problems or making decisions, fatigue, and feeling irritable or overwhelmed. You can start a stress management program to help you get through those difficult situations and not develop the serious problems we mentioned above.

Seeing what stress can do to people, it is imperative to learn how to develop the ability to be resilient when we face stress related situations and changes that can generate this response. The Latin word "resilio" is where the word resilience stems from and it means to retaliate. So, resilience is the way we hold ourselves to tackle the problems we face and move on from them as a stronger person. There are three parts of emotional resilience on which we can start building on this important skill. There is the physical element, which translates into good health, energy, and physical strength. There is the psychological element that has to do with self-confidence, self-expression,- self-esteem, and good thinking abilities and last we have the social relationships you have and how healthy they are, for example, are they based on communication and cooperation?

Emotional resilience is not a new concept to adults since this is something we are born with. For example, some people are not at all affected by changes that are not programmed and others cannot stand them. Also, emotional resilience can be affected by your age, gender, and whether or not you have experienced a past traumatic experience. The great thing about emotional resilience is that it is not a skill you can or cannot have. There are many levels to master and even if you manage to not develop emotional resilience to its fullest, still you will have done an amazing job and your life easier.

In many resilience training programs those levels that need to be conquered are taught with the endgame being for someone to achieve emotional awareness. To start with, one of the main characteristics and first step in your journey to be emotionally resilient is self-awareness. Self-awareness is the ability to acknowledge and be in tune with your own feelings, as well as possible inside conflicts that you have developed. Through your journey to achieve self-awareness, you will be able to understand better to what extent your feelings are responsible for your actions rather than throwing the blame to other or environmental factors. You will learn how to look for all the necessary answers inside yourself and take responsibility for your actions.

By practicing self-awareness, you will notice that your relationships will be better since you will finally be clear and certain about your needs and what you want. Your moods will also get better since it is extremely depended on your emotions and how you choose to think about yourself. As you become more self-aware, you will learn how to listen to your body, thoughts, emotion, and behavior as well as the relationship that exists between those four factors. You will communicate more effectively since you will get a better understanding of what you believe in and your decision making skills will develop more because many bad choices we make are the result of thinking when we were emotionally charged.

To develop self-awareness are a few steps that you need to follow and watch out for. One thing you could do is to notice the things that bother you on other people. This will help you actually pinpoint some of the habits that are bothering you about yourself since it is often pointed out by experts that some of the things that irritate us in other people are nothing more but a reflection of something we don't like about our appearance or personality. For example, that may be placing the needs of others ahead of our own or avoiding conflict even though we are right about something.

Another way that will help you developing self-awareness is the mindfulness meditation techniques we analyzed in previous chapters to learn more about your emotions as well as your body. Also, you need to watch out for not paying too much attention to details or think too much out of a situation that is not that important or affects you immediately. Added to this, you need to also identify the triggers that cause you unwanted emotions such as prolonged sadness, anxiety or shame about yourself.

For example, you may feel anxious or angry during social gatherings because you are afraid of other people judging you about your views, looks, and even on how much you drink. You may find out that before you identified the trigger that is causing you such emotions, you were going to extreme lengths to avoid this trigger and distract yourself. The point of self-awareness and at the end of emotional resilience is to identify the problems you have with yourself and fixing them so as to be able to endure the stress and changes that will occur throughout your life.

Also, you could ask your friends and family to give you some feedback on yourself. Nobody is perfect and sometimes we are not able to pinpoint the parts of our personality that needs extra work. However, the people that love may notice those parts as you are noticing theirs. Ask someone that loves you about those blind spots you are not able to see and try to work to make them better. Maybe you are not a very patient person or you are not expressing your needs and your emotions to the point of letting other people impose their beliefs on you. Fixing those blind spots will make you become more self-aware and emotionally resilient throughout your life.

By knowing your weaknesses as well as your strengths, you will be able to work on those things that keep you from reaching your goals and make you less self-aware and emotionally resilient. Set boundaries that will help you maintain your goal and not make you lose the progress you have made in being more self-aware. Understanding what your limits are is an integral part of self-awareness and at the end of conquering emotional resilience.

Persistence combined with the motivation to achieve your goals whether they are making your dreams come true or obtaining emotional resilience. Persistence helps a person develop the consistency needed to deal with external stressors as well as handling internal emotional conflicts, thus making him or her emotionally resilient. Self-control will also help you when you are trying to gain emotional resilience. People who have emotional self-control are able to harness their feelings and redirect them to a more productive activity, so they will be less affected by stress and will not let it affect their lives as much as other people let it affect them.

Emotional self-control is the skill many people have developed to manage the emotions that disturb them and remain productive, even when they are under stress and have to deal with situations that would cause other people to fret. To develop your emotional self-control, you should first let a small amount of time pass between your emotions and response to them. It may not always be easy to manage your emotions; however, you can control your response to them. Pause for a moment and let yourself think before you act on what you feel. If there is no need for you to respond immediately, then let yourself think and calm for twenty-four hours. Also, you should wait before passing emotional judgment until you are certain you have all the facts. Making assumptions about something when the information we have is limited may lead us to say the wrong thing or making a big mistake we may not be able to fix later on.

Optimism will also help you on your journey of developing your emotional resilience since when we see the positive aspect even in the most stressful situations; we are able to cope with them in a more effective manner. It is often noted that people who have strong emotional resilience are able to laugh at the difficulties they may face because it can prevent you from facing those difficulties as a threat and therefore change the way your body will respond to stress. Being optimistic and having a great sense of humor about life's tough times can be a life altering move in both a physical as well as an emotional level. But what are the characteristics of people with strong emotional resilience skills?

People who have developed their emotional resilience are aware of every situation they find themselves in, their emotional reactions, and how people around are behaving. They know that in order to handle their emotions, they have to know what is causing them as well as the reason why they are caused. They are aware, resilient, and able to maintain control even in difficult situations by finding new ways to deal with current or future problems. They understand that life is full of changes and challenges and that people cannot avoid every problem. What they can do is to be open-minded and able to adapt to changes.

They know how to practice a considerable amount of control over their own lives by not blaming others for their problems and mistakes. They know that every problem or mistake they make is theirs to deal with and do not depend much on others to offer them a solution, and even if they ask for a second opinion, they will act as they deem fit because they know that any action they take will affect the result of an event and it will also affect them. Even if our problems are caused by external factors, it is important to know that we have the power necessary to choose what to do next and that these choices will affect our current state, our coping abilities as well as the future.

People who have developed emotional resilience have problem-solving skills that are essential for handling crises since with those skills, resilient people are able to find the solution that has the least dangerous outcome. When most people are going through a stressful and dangerous situation, they fail to notice important details and take advantage of potential opportunities that may be provided in order not only to solve the problem but avoid future similar situations too. Problem-solving skills are an essential part of developing emotional resilience and the ability everyone should develop even kids and teenagers. For adult problem-solving skills will help them make better decisions and learn how to be more aware of a difficult situation without having to resort to stress and fear, waiting for the situation to pass.

So what should you do to enhance and develop your problem-solving skills? To start with you should focus on the solution and on the problem you face at the moment. It is pretty simple as a step and the explanation behind it is just as simple. You cannot let your brain think of solutions when you turn your whole attention on the problem. When you focus on the problem instead of the solution, you are feeding yourself with negativity which in turn is translated to negative emotions.

Those negative emotions are responsible for you not being able to find potential solutions. Acknowledge the problem and try to remain calm. Then try to focus on the possible way you can deal with the problem instead of overanalyzing while wondering whose fault was that or what went wrong. As soon as you have dealt with the problem effectively, you will be able to pose those questions and prevent the same problem from happening twice.

You can take it a step further and change the way you think about problems. Most people don't want to deal with a situation that is overwhelming, irritating, and seems impossible to solve at first. However, if you decide to view those problems as a way to grow or as a challenge that will make you stronger, you will be less stressed about finding the needed solution. You will let your brain focus and break down the problem to analyze it in an easier way making you more flexible to deal with it and training you to solve future problems the same way. Your problems are opportunities to grow as a person they are lessons you need to be taught to protect from future hurt and pain.

You should also understand that not all problems are worth stressing over. For example, if your car doesn't start in the morning there is an obvious solution to that problem. Make a list of problems that have an actual negative impact on you and call them worst-case scenarios. Minor setbacks are not the end of the world and everything is happening to teach us something. If we take the example of your car not starting, next time you may think that you have to start a bit earlier for work than usual to catch a bus or the train if something like this happens again. This is a lesson you were taught because of a minor setback.

When you are facing a problem, simplify it by removing all the details. Go to the core of the problem. This way you will be able to find out the simplest and obvious solution to the problem that may have eluded you due to all the details you had to think of and maybe they weren't necessary to build your solution. It could also help to note as many solutions as possible for each problem, even the ones that you deem as ridiculous. With problem-solving, keeping an open mind is the very first element of finding the appropriate solution. Ridiculous solutions may lead you to the perfect one or even a ridiculous solution may be the one that needs to be adopted so as to solve the problem that is troubling you.

With each solution, you come up with, brainstorm the potential results both positive and negative. When you are finished doing this for each solution, choose the one that has a less negative impact according to your standards. If the choice you made was the wrong one, there is no need to beat yourself up about it. Embrace your mistakes and learn from them.

Problem-solving is not about getting always positive results. It's about solving your problems and even when choose the wrong solution, you are able to learn from it and apply your developed problem-solving skills more effectively next time. Also, if you another chance to fix the application of the wrong solution go back to choose a different one from the list you have made or make a new list of the positive and negative outcomes from each solution, using the new data you gathered from applying the first solution.

Apart from problem-solving skills, resilient people have a strong social circle that includes friends and family. Resilient people know the importance of support and have surrounded themselves with people that truly love them and would help them without aiming for any personal gain or having feelings of jealousy. Everyone that is close to resilient people truly cares about them and wish to see them succeed because a person who is resilient knows exactly what he or she needs and what they can offer to others.

They see themselves as survivors and not as a victim of a situation. Victimizing yourself will only make you depressed and lack any motivation for solving the problem at hand. Resilient people know that and by viewing themselves as survivors they are focusing on solving the challenges with determination, even when the situation seems impossible to solve. They are focused on attaining the most positive outcome given the circumstances, and there are many times they succeed in solving a problem effectively.

Another characteristic of resilient people is seeking assistance not only from people but from other sources too. For example, they read books about people who have gone through the same problems as them and how they managed to deal with it. They enrich themselves with the necessary knowledge to deal with any predictable or unpredictable challenged. When things get too rough for them, they join support groups to find people that are facing the same challenges as them and know how to provide the necessary support and compassion.

Enhance your resilience by finding a purpose in your life. There is no greater motivation to tackle any problems or challenges than to attain your life's purpose. Your mindset will immediately change and view those problems as lessons you need to be taught, especially if your goal and purpose are desirable enough for you. Trusting in your abilities and viewing them in a positive way is also a great way to develop your resilience. Have confidence in your ability to cope with stressful situations and to do that you need to start working on enhancing your self-esteem. Your strengths and accomplishments will be your tools and guide with which you will succeed in life.

To be resilient, you should be flexible and able to adapt to change. Embrace change and see them as an opportunity to learn new things and move your life to a new path. If everything stayed the same, people would be bored and not able to challenge themselves to becoming the best version of themselves. Understand that there will be setbacks on the road and view them with as much optimism as you can muster given the circumstances. There will be difficult times, but when those times are over, a brighter future will come and you will have the tools necessary to cope or even avoid a similar situation.

When you are faced with a difficult situation, it is easy to forget to take care of yourself. You may end up losing your appetite or eat too much, neglect exercising, not get enough sleep, and all these will come as a reaction to dealing with stress. Try to indulge in activities that make you feel good and loved. Even the simplest things can better your mood and let us not forget that self-care is an extremely important process to follow when you are building your emotional resilience. If you are not feeling good about yourself, you will not be able to control your emotions as effectively as you would under different circumstances.

Self-care may include you taking a relaxing bath filled with essential oils and scented soaps or nourishing your skin. You will have to follow a healthy diet and exercise regularly for your body to be prepared to face the stress levels associated with a difficult situation. If your body suffers, your mind will suffer too and by extent, your emotional resilience will not work.

When we wait for a problematic situation to pass without taking any action, we are only succeeding in prolonging the crisis. If you will not take immediate action to solve a challenge, you will end up being more stressed and never manage to find an effective solution to a problem that otherwise may have a simple way out. Whether or not the problem you are facing has a simple solution, you should focus on the progress you have made so far and plan your next move. This will keep you from being discouraged by everything that needs to be done until the problem is over. Keep working on the skills you have developed to achieve the emotional resilience needed for you to face your problems. When you find yourself lacking motivation, think of how your life will be much better the moment you will resolve the situation effectively.

Most resilient people face their fears straight on since this is the only way to deal with them effectively. When you avoid the things that scare you, they will make you more scared and the time will come when you will be forced to deal with them. It would be better for you to face them at the time you choose and you will be ready than to be forced to face them when you are not prepared and may make rash decisions. When you are forced and rushed into making a decision, chances are you will end up making a mistake. This is why emotionally resilient people face their fears from the start to avoid situations that will force them to make a mistake with severe implications for their future.

Appreciate what you have in your life and show gratitude towards other people and to yourself. You will be more resilient than ever before if you focus on the things you have accomplished rather than complain about the different choices you could have made or the things that you lost because you didn't follow a certain path or grabbed an opportunity at the appropriate time. Every choice we make opens a new path on which we should adapt and make the best of it. You can always change the things you don't like and resilient people know this. Instead of feeling depressed and complain about the things you weren't able to do, stop, make a plan, and make those dreams happen.

Making a list of your accomplishments and everything that you should be grateful for will help you develop this mindset and as time passes, this practice will be done automatically by you. For example you can make a weekly plan including a series of things to be grateful for such as things that you have that other people are not so fortunate to have, three goals you have set and accomplished during this week, three people that made you happy this week, six good things that happened to you this week, six things that you should be grateful to your family for, and what goals you would like to set for the plan of the next week.

By replacing negative thoughts with positive ones and maintaining a healthy lifestyle, you will see many things change during the course of your life. Be open to accepting criticism since this is the way for you to pinpoint your weak points and work on them. If you feel that there is nothing important in your life to challenge you and practice being resilient on, take up a new hobby or learn a new skill. It is extremely important for people to spend time with their family and friends. Resilient people have emotions too and a hard situation can affect them a lot, even though they refuse to give up. By spending time with the people you love and love you in return, you will be able to forget for a while the problems you are facing and focus on spending enjoyable moments that seem as a delightful break from the everyday stress.

It is a widely known fact that stress will affect your body and your ability to listen to it will suffer a considerable blow if you are not able to handle it. Emotional resilience will protect you and the progress you have made while trying to listen to your body, from having to start all over again. Apart from this emotional resilience, will help you be more aware of your potential and your emotions, therefore you will know how these emotions turn into a physical reaction. Searching for the different ways to deal with the problem at hand will only make you stronger, so don't forget to practice your problem-solving skills too.

Chapter 7: Develop Your Self-Regulation

Self-regulation is the final important skill we are going to analyze when it comes to handling your emotions, your stress levels, and therefore being free to listen to your body. As adults we are able to pretty much do everything we want at any time we want as long as we are within logical boundaries and we don't harm others. For example, we don't need to go to work every day, the vast majority of people will go to jail for skipping a day or two from work. Or we can eat cake or pizza for breakfast if that is what we desire. So, why are we going to work every day and why we prefer to eat pizza or cake for breakfast? How do we force ourselves to endure working on a day that this is the last place we would like to be in? How do we keep ourselves from not indulging in an unhealthy breakfast and we go for the healthy choice?

To the above questions, the answer is self-regulation, a process that most people follow without even thinking this is what they are practicing at a precise moment. Self-regulation is a skill that has to do with controlling our emotions, behaviors, and thoughts in favor of achieving the goals we have set for the future. This is why we are able to control our impulses of not going to work or eating an unhealthy breakfast. In other words, we are taught to think before we act, we practice self-control. A person who has developed self-regulation skills can keep his or her emotions under control and resist indulging in impulsive behaviors that might end up harming them. They can also cheer themselves up whenever they are feeling down and they can also match their emotional as well as their behavioral responses to the demands of their environment.

The ability to self-regulate in adulthood comes from our childhood since it is an important skill, children need to be taught for their emotional maturity and their future social interactions as they grow to be adults. Emotional self-regulation is the ability of a person to control or influence his or her emotions by taking the necessary steps to get himself or herself out of a bad mood or destress. Behavioral self-regulation is the ability of a person to act on behalf of his or her long-term goal and interests in a wat that is connected with his or her values. For example, you may not want to go to work, but you decide to go because you need money to live and know that it will reflect badly on your future goals if you aim for a promotion or to put some money aside to make your dreams happen.

Self-regulation will help both a child and an adult to control his or her cognitive impulses to respond to an uncomfortable feeling or environmental threats. For example, as a child, you may have been prone to throwing tantrums and grown into an adult who has learned how to tolerate the emotions that made you uncomfortable without having to resort to the behavior you had adopted as a child. Now, you are able to control your urges to act on emotions that make you uncomfortable and trigger a response that you have deemed as bad.

Self-regulation is a process in which we must be cautious of our behavior, the things that influence it as well as the consequences our behavior has on ourselves and our surroundings. Values are extremely important because we must judge our behavior according to our own standards as well as the standards presented by our broader environment. Also, we must ponder sometimes about what we think of our own behavior and the different ways we deal when faced with an important situation or decision. Do we often give in to our impulses? Do we let our emotions control our behavior which often leads us to make many mistakes?

In other words, you should take a pause and take some time between what you feel and your actions. Taking the necessary time between those two will let you think everything you are dealing with through, form a plan, and wait until your plan can be executed and wait for the results to become apparent. Children, as well as adults, may not find those steps easy to follow, but the problems caused by lacking the self-regulation skills will make anyone who wants to better his or her life develop them.

For example, a child who does not practice self-regulation will give in to his or her anger and may even resort to hitting other children out of frustration and that, in turn, will make him less able to maintain friendships and will face reprimands from his or her school. Most children resort to bullying due to this fact. They are not able to control their emotions that correspond to actions along with other psychological problems they may face. As far as children are concerned, they must be taught self-regulation skills or they are going to face many difficulties in their adult lives with behaviors that are developed from childhood.

Many adults suffer from poor self-regulation skills and self-confidence because they weren't taught as children how to develop those necessary abilities. Adults who lack those skills will have trouble handling stress and their anger. They are more prone to developing a mental disorder and they will develop anxiety disorders due to the fact that they will not be able to control their anger and other emotions such as sadness and fear. They may not even have a developed value system that would allow them to act according to it and they will have trouble expressing themselves appropriately. For example, if an adult values achieving in academics, he or she will not let themselves slack off before a test, in contrast to someone who will do so if he hasn't learned self-regulation.

So, people face problems with self-regulation because their childhood was not ideal. He or she may have felt insecure and not as safe as they should. In other cases, where self-regulation problems were not caused by problematic childhood, the adult may not have followed the necessary strategies for managing feelings that would have made him or her uncomfortable. Self-regulation and self-control have a lot in common since they are very similar concepts. However, according to psychologist Stuart Shanker, they differ on two basic matters:

"Self-control is about inhibiting strong impulses; self-regulation is about reducing the frequency and intensity of strong impulses by managing stress-load and recovery. In fact, self-regulation is what makes self-control possible, or, in many cases, unnecessary."

Self-regulation is a more automatic process that happens in our subconscious unless a person chooses to monitor his or her behavior and feeling to control the self-regulation process. To further understand the concept of self-regulation, it is better to see what happens in action. Let us take a cashier who successfully remains calm and polite when he or she is berated from an angry customer for a situation he or she has no control over. Another example can be that of a child who does not throw a tantrum when he or she is told by the parents that he or she cannot have the desirable toy. A couple who is arguing about something important and decide to take some time to cool off can be another example of practicing self-regulation.

When it comes to listening to your body, an appropriate example can be when you are trying to lose weight in order for you to be the best, healthier part of yourself, and you go out with a friend at a restaurant. While your friend may eat everything he or she wants, you decide to stick with the healthier choice because you know that eating unhealthy food will push back and affect your goals.

What can you do though to develop your self-regulation abilities? The first thing you can do and we have already analyzed is practicing mindfulness. With mindfulness, you will be able to place some distance between your emotions and reactions and focus on relaxation and calmness. Another strategy you can follow and will allow you to enhance your self-regulation abilities is cognitive reappraisal or else cognitive reframing. Cognitive reappraisal includes changing your mindset, in other words, the way you think about things. To be more specific, during this method you will have to interpret again a difficult and stressful situation you had to endure in order to alter your emotional response to it.

An example of such a case can be the fact that your good friend had not contacted you in days or even does not return your texts and calls. That will make you feel neglected and you will probably stress about him or her avoiding you or that he or she doesn't want to speak with you ever again. With cognitive reappraisal, you will think that your friend may be really busy or is facing a problem with his or her own, instead of thinking that your friend hates you. If you practice cognitive reappraisal in your everyday life, you will be able to replace any negative emotions with positive ones and change your mindset for the better.

Some other effective strategies for self-regulation are acceptance of a situation and problem-solving skills, instead of avoidance, distraction, worrying, and suppression of emotions. The first step to self-regulation is to accept and recognize that people have a choice on how to react to every situation they face. More specifically, you have three options that include avoidance, attack, and approach. It is a fact that your feelings will lead to one path, but the truth is that you are not forced to listen to your feelings every time. You have control over them and behaving in a certain manner is your choice.

Then, you should monitor your body since this is the one which will give you the necessary clues about how you are feeling, especially in cases that your feelings are not apparent to you. For example, when your heart beats rapidly this may be a sign that you are entering a rage state or you are going through a panic attack. You should ask yourself if you are running away from difficult situations constantly. What are your emotions and your body's response during that time? Do you feel the need to scream in anger at someone who has hurt you or done something wrong? Will you get anything out of screaming your anger out or should you discuss the situation when you are calm? Start with building your boundaries and your value system rather than trying to suppress emotions. Try to see the larger picture and act in a way that will benefit you and the people around you.

Self-regulation is an integral part of emotional intelligence. According to Mayer's and Salovey's model of emotional intelligence, this ability is defined as:

"The ability to perceive emotions, to access and generate emotions so as to assist thought, to understand emotions and emotional knowledge, and to reflectively regulate emotions so as to promote emotional and intellectual growth"

According to expert Daniel Goleman, emotional intelligence is consisted of three parts, which are self-awareness, empathy, self-regulation, social skills, and internal motivation. Self-regulation, the ability to control or influence our emotions, is an essential part of emotional intelligence because the better we can understand and face our emotions and those of others, the better we will become to understanding the environment we find ourselves in and adapt to this environment which will result in pursuing our goals in a much easier way than before.

Usually, adults have problems practicing self-regulation at work because they are not able to handle their emotions under pressure. To better manage your emotions at work, you should do some breathing exercises; stay hydrated by drinking lots of water, eating healthy, and sleep at least eight hours a night. When you are trying to practice self-regulation, you should keep in mind some pointers that will help you succeed.

You should try to live your life with integrity by being a good role model for your family, friends, and to everyone, you associate yourself with. Live by the values you have adopted and try not to bend them for anyone. Be open to change and challenge yourself to deal with it in the best way that you can. If you find yourself struggling, work to improve your adaptation abilities and stay positive that you will succeed.

Identify what triggers certain behaviors by being aware of your strengths and weaknesses as well as what your limits are. When you pinpoint the triggers responsible for your bad behavior, try to change those behaviors by practicing meditation to stay focused and calm. Self-discipline is important when you want to achieve self-regulation. Work persistently towards your goals and that includes not reacting badly to every difficult situation you may face. If you react according to your emotions every time, you will face extreme setbacks that will make you lose any motivation to become what you always wished to be.

Take a step back from your thoughts and try to tackle the negative emotions associated with them, but never ignore your thoughts. Acknowledge them, analyze them, and try to solve the problems that are causing them. Letting go of negativity will open many opportunities for you and your mind will be clear to tackle effectively any task you will be given.

You will be able to think more clearly if you detach yourself from difficult situations and keep calm when you are asked to solve a problem. You will be able to consider the consequences of your actions. For example, what would happen if you did not follow self-regulation on a pressing matter and gave in to anger and frustration? Would the results of each course of action be different or would they remain the same? Keep in mind that there are also long-term consequences to your choices that will affect your future. If you keep thinking of this, you will be able to place some distance between your emotions and your actions.

Believing in yourself is the base of all self-regulation practices. You will need to work on your self-confidence and focus on your successes in life instead of pondering on your mistakes. Embrace failure, even though it is hard for many people to do so. Fear of failure is the most important reason why many people do not try to do the things they want because they are afraid of making a fool of themselves. However, if you think that challenging ourselves will help strengthen us and learn from both our success stories and failures, you will be ready to embark on any journey you wish to without having to worry about the ending.

By embracing your mistakes you will take out the fear factor and be free to make your choices in accordance with your problem-solving skills. Challenging yourself little by little on a regular basis will help you built your confidence and personality. You could start by learning a new skill or taking up the hobby you wished to do for so long. Do everything in your power to succeed in both the skill and hobby you love. Push your limits a little more every time and enhance your curiosity about what will happen when you succeed. If you do not succeed, you will gain the necessary knowledge and insight to try again and this time avoid the mistakes you did previously.

Listening to our bodies will be an easy thing to do by following everything we have analyzed so far. Before you start practicing the methods that will enable you to succeed in this goal you have set, you should always keep in mind that positivity is the right perspective of which we should view life. Negativity never helped anyone and caused harm to the people who decided to give in to it. According to Kendra Cherry, author of Very Well Mind, the definition of positivity is,

"Positive thinking actually means approaching life's challenges with a positive outlook. It does not necessarily mean avoiding or ignoring the bad things; instead, it involves making the most of the

potentially bad situations, trying to see the best in other people, and viewing yourself and your abilities in a positive light."

So, acknowledge that bit everything in life will go as you have planned them and be willing to make any effort necessary to realize your dreams even if you don't think they will pay off. Appreciate the good things life has to offer and grasp the opportunity you are given to develop a connection with your body. Do not forget that a positive attitude is considered the key to success because if you give in to pessimism and negativity you are surrendering your control to your emotions and will wallow in misery since you will be missing out an important opportunity you are given in leading a happy life through growth and development.

You want your body to respond to the connection you are trying to build with it in a positive way that will help you remain healthy for many years to come. If you approach this connection while maintaining negative emotions, it may as well shut you out and take the cue from you and be less resilient and strong. Optimism when forging a connection with your body will reduce the chances of you developing depression and high levels of stress as well as bring you the happiness so many people crave to attain.

Conclusion

Listening to your body is not as easy or as hard as everyone would like to think. The truth is that no one ever told us as we were growing up how to listen and communicate with the only thing that we should take care of to be healthy, happy, and free to act however you would like. We were taught only to listen to other people who knew better what our bodies want and we started reading stuff that was harming us by not only making us start counting calories, it made us also eat in ways that not enough energy was provided and as a result, someone may have felt tired all day long.

We need to stop trying to be thin and start listening to our bodies. The means to get thin, if they come from the wrong source, will make your body struggle to get all the nutrients it needs. The human body needs certain quantities of nutrients to function properly and only each body knows what is healthy for it and what is not. Embrace your body for all its faults and beauty and most of all respect it. Replace any possible negative thoughts you have of it with thoughts about being grateful to it for the way it works, for the way it keeps you protected and helps you function throughout the day.

Practice meditation and exercises we have analyzed throughout the course of this book to help you connect to your body and mind. If you find yourself be skeptical about those practices, place a hand over your heart and feel it beat rhythmically. As you focus on that sound, close your eyes and try to feel the response of your body at the attention you are giving it. This will make you realize how important it is to start caring for the one thing that encompasses the reason you are alive.

Try to figure out what your body needs to stay healthy from now on. Maybe you need to exercise it, maybe you even need a new mattress to help you get a better night's sleep and relax it as much as you can. Taking small steps will help you stay committed to your goal. Find one thing at a time that your body needs and try to fix that before moving on to the next. For example, eat only when you feel hungry and not because it is time to eat. You might be comfortable eating six meals instead of three, and there is nothing wrong with that. Go with the flow, your body needs you to.

Also, no one is telling you that it is wrong to snack, but instead of eating chips every day, you could buy vegetables, fruit or crackers and have a healthy snack. You can eat everything with moderation. Your body is not able to process a whole cake no matter how good it tastes and makes you feel. Try eating small portions of each food that you crave in order for your body to be able to process it. Do not let your feelings dictate the way you eat and take care of your body. Think of the food as the fuel you are giving to your car, you want your car to be given the best quality of fuel because it may develop serious functional problems in the future if given the lowest quality possible.

We are listening to our bodies when we are thirsty or want to go to the bathroom or when it needs sleep. It is not that hard to do that with other functions of our body. Keep in mind the skills needed to learn on how to listen to your body will take time to develop and practice as it happens with every other skill we decide to develop. If you find it hard keeping up with the cues your body is sending you, you could even start a journal and write about them.

Living in a noisy and stressful environment will make it harder to achieve this goal. Most people know they have to take care of their bodies, but they do not have the time. If you realize the importance and the benefits of being able to listen to your body and take care of it, you will realize that time is something you will be able to make for such an important task. So, be aware of the sensations and the cues your body is sending you to achieve a healthy lifestyle that will empower you to live with the best version of yourself.

Bibliography

1. Dr. Belinda Hollis: Stranded brain Introduction to Neuro Linguistic Programming, October 2019

2. Lise Bourbeau: EGO: The Greatest Obstacle to Healing the 5 Wounds, May 15, 2017.

3. Thich Nhat Hanh: Making Space: Creating a Home Meditation Practice, November 3, 2011.

4. Shunryu Suzuki: Zen Mind, Beginner's Mind: Informal Talks on Zen Meditation and Practice, June 28, 2011.

5. Dan Harris: 10% Happier: How I Tamed the Voice in My Head, Reduced Stress Without Losing My Edge, and Found Self-Help That Actually Works--A True Story, December 30, 2014.

6. Bhante Henepola Gunaratana: Mindfulness in Plain English, September 6, 2011.

7. Dr. Harry Barry: Emotional Resilience: How to safeguard your mental health (The Flag Series), 3 May 2018.

8. Geetu Bharwaney: Emotional Resilience: Know What it Takes to be Agile, Adaptable & Perform at Your Best, May 26, 2015.

9. Mark Williams and Danny Penman: Mindfulness: An Eight-Week Plan for Finding Peace in a Frantic World, November 13, 2012.

10. Matthew Sockolov: Practicing Mindfulness: 75 Essential Meditations to Reduce Stress, Improve Mental Health, and Find Peace in the Everyday, September 11, 2018.

11. Rohan Gunatillake: Mindfulness Cards: Simple Practices for Everyday Life (Daily Mindfulness, Daily Gratitude, Mindful Meditation), April 10, 2018.

12. Lori Jean Glass: #HealthyAdult: PIVOT from Fantasy to Reality, Confusion to Clarity, Isolation to Connection, May 28, 2019.

13. Wendy Suzuki and Billie Fitzpatrick: Healthy Brain, Happy Life: A Personal Program to Activate Your Brain and Do Everything Better, May 19, 2015.

14. Alice Boyes: The Healthy Mind Toolkit: Simple Strategies to Get Out of Your Own Way and Enjoy Your Life, May 1, 2018.

15. Samantha Harris: Your Healthiest Healthy: 8 Easy Ways to Take Control, Help Prevent and Fight Cancer, and Live a Longer, Cleaner, Happier Life, September 18, 2018.

www.ingramcontent.com/pod-product-compliance
Lightning Source LLC
Chambersburg PA
CBHW060323030426

42336CB00011B/1184